D1118758

Understanding Psychiatric Treatment

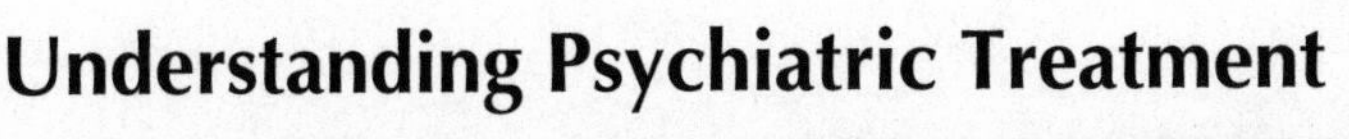

Understanding Psychiatric Treatment

Therapy for Serious Mental Health Disorder in Adults

Edited by

Gerald O'Mahony
St Bartholomew's Hospital, University of London

and

James V. Lucey
St Bartholomew's Hospital, University of London

JOHN WILEY & SONS
Chichester · New York · Weinheim · Brisbane · Singapore · Toronto

Baffins Lane, Chichester,
West Sussex PO19 1UD, England

National 01243 779777
International (+44) 1243 779777
e-mail (for orders and customer service enquiries):
cs-books@wiley.co.uk
Visit our Home Page on http://www.wiley.co.uk
or http://www.wiley.com

Other Wiley Editorial Offices

John Wiley & Sons, Inc., 605 Third Avenue,
New York, NY 10158-0012, USA

Wiley-VCH Verlag, GmbH,
Pappelallee 3, D-69469 Weinheim, Germany

Jacaranda Wiley Ltd, 33 Park Road, Milton,
Queensland 4064, Australia

John Wiley & Sons (Asia) Ptd Ltd, 2 Clementi Loop #02-01,
Jin Xing Distripark, Singapore 129809

John Wiley & Sons (Canada) Ltd, 22 Worcester Road,
Rexdale, Ontario M9W 1LI, Canada

Library of Congress Cataloging-in-Publication Data

Understanding psychiatric treatment : therapy for serious mental health disorders in adults / edited by Gerald O'Mahony, James V. Lucey.
p. cm.
Includes bibliographical references and index.
ISBN 0-471-97570-2 (paper : alk. paper)
1. Mental illness—Treatment. 2. Mentally ill—Medical care.
I. O'Mahony, Gerald. II. Lucey, James V.
[DNLM: 1. Mental Disorders—therapy. 2. Psychotherapy—methods.
WM 400 U55 1998]
RC480.U53 1998
616.89'1—dc21
DNLM/DLC
for Library of Congress 97-43723
CIP

British Library Cataloguing in Publication Data

A catalogue record for this book is available from the British Library

ISBN 0-471-97570-2

Typeset in 11/13pt Palatino by Dorwyn Ltd, Rowlands Castle, Hampshire
Printed and bound in Great Britain by Biddles Ltd, Guildford and Kings Lynn
This book is printed on acid-free paper responsibly manufactured from sustainable forestry, in which at least two trees are planted for each one used for paper production.

Contents

About the Editors

Dr Gerald O'Mahony is a Consultant Psychiatrist at St Bartholomew's and Homerton Hospital working with the elderly in East London. He qualified in Medicine at the National University of Ireland, University College Cork, in 1977. He worked in general practice in South Wales, and medicine in Southern Africa, before training in psychiatry in Dublin and Cardiff. His clinical interests are in psychiatry as allied to medicine. He is married to Mary, a general practitioner, and has three children.

Dr James V. Lucey is a Consultant Psychiatrist/Senior Lecturer at St Bartholomew's and Homerton Hospital where he is responsible for the psychiatric intensive care unit and the anxiety disorders clinic. He qualified in medicine at the Royal College of Surgeons, National University of Ireland in 1983 and later trained in psychiatry at St Patrick's Hospital, Dublin, and the Maudsley Hospital, London. His research interests include the management of severe anxiety disorders and their biology. He is married to Philippine and has three children.

List of Contributors

Dr Dinesh Bhugra .... Senior Lecturer, Institute of Psychiatry, De Crespigny Park, Denmark Hill, London SE5 8AF

Dr Kamaldeep Bhui .... Institute of Psychiatry, De Crespigny Park, Denmark Hill, London SE5 8AF

Professor T.G. Dinan .... Chairman, Department of Psychiatry, Royal College of Surgeons in Ireland, Dublin

Dr Sandra Evans .... Senior Lecturer, Department of Psychological Medicine, St Bartholomew's Hospital, West Smithfield, London EC1A 7BE

Dr David Healy .... Senior Lecturer, Division of Psychological Medicine, University of Wales College of Medicine, Bangor, Gwynedd LL57 2PW

Professor Robert W. Kerwin .. Head of Section of Clinical Neuropharmacology, Institute of Psychiatry, De Crespigny Park, Denmark Hill, London SE5 8AF

Dr James V. Lucey .... Senior Lecturer, Department of Psychological Medicine, St Bartholomew's Hospital, West Smithfield, London EC1A 7BE

Dr Kevin Lynch .... c/o Professor Kerwin, Institute of Psychiatry, De Crespigny Park, Denmark Hill, London SE5 8AF

Dr Tom McMonagle .... Lecturer, Division of Psychological Medicine, University of Wales College of Medicine, Bangor, Gwynedd LL57 2PW

Professor Anne Mortimer .... c/o Professor Kerwin, Institute of Psychiatry, De Crespigny Park, Denmark Hill, London SE5 8AF

Dr Siobhan Murphy .... Senior Lecturer, Department of Psychological Medicine, St Bartholomew's Hospital, West Smithfield, London EC1A 7BE

Dr Anne-Marie O'Dwyer .... Hon Lecturer, Psychological Treatment Unit, Maudsley Hospital, Denmark Hill, London SE5 8AF

Dr Gerald O'Mahony .... Consultant Psychiatrist, Department of Psychological Medicine, St Bartholomew's Hospital, West Smithfield, London EC1A 7BE

Dr Michael J. Travis .... Research Psychiatrist, Institute of Psychiatry, Institute of Psychiatry, De Crespigny Park, Denmark Hill, London SE5 8AF

Foreword

Anthony W. Clare

We live at a time when tried and tested treatments jostle with alternative or complementary therapies which have never been tested and which are more often than not touted as panaceas for all manner of diseases. Contemporary psychiatry does possess proven treatments, yet there is still considerable scepticism concerning their effectiveness. Paradoxically, there is a heady enthusiasm and substantial appetite for all sorts of alternative therapies – herbal remedies, vitamin supplements, acupuncture, homeopathy, massage, reflexology, and a plethora of interventions variously described as 'psychotherapies' – some of which have never been subjected to properly controlled scientific trials and for which there is no substantial evidence of effectiveness.

Within medicine as much as outside it, psychiatry's reputation remains that of a domain in which speculative theories of causation are as numerous as effective therapies are scarce. Yet it is a measure of how much progress has been made that today one of the several challenges facing psychiatry is how best to integrate the expanding knowledge of biological, psychological and social factors in psychiatric illness so as to ensure that the wide range of available treatments are appropriately and efficiently deployed. Hitherto, psychiatry has been a fissiparous and argumentative discipline. Proponents of the psychotherapies, social model theorists and biologically inclined enthusiasts have warred with each other with all the dogmatic intolerance and monoptic vision of religious zealots. While there has been and there still is much talk of 'bio-psycho-social' approaches and 'holistic' treatment, one of the most persistent criticisms to be heard about contemporary psychiatric practitioners is that they are blinkered in their devotion to this or that therapeutic school and indifferent to any other.

It is not easy to find a readable, fair, dispassionate and useful account, not merely of the available effective treatments in modern psychiatry but of how they are believed to exercise their effects. The eclectic approach has never exerted as potent an appeal as the ideologically biased. Thus to find within the same text a judicious account of the scientific status of electroconvulsive therapy and a balanced overview of the role of group psychotherapy is not just novel and refreshing, it is vital if psychiatry is to progress and if patients are to be provided with as wide a range of appropriate and effective treatments as possible. Perhaps the real significance of this book, however, is the testimony it bears to the fruitful developments that have occurred in psychiatric therapy over the past twenty years. During that period there has been the introduction of the selective serotonin reuptake group of drugs, the deployment of newer and more effective so-called 'atypical' antipsychotic drugs in schizophrenia, the identification of the effective elements in the cognitive and other behavioural forms of psychotherapy and the clarification of the role played by social factors such as unemployment and poverty in the cause and course of the major psychiatric conditions.

Notwithstanding these and other advances, there remain controversial issues within the field of psychiatric therapy. For example, while the ability of psychiatrists to treat acute episodes of various illnesses including manic depression, schizophrenia, anorexia nervosa, obsessive compulsive disorder and phobic anxiety is in many instances impressive, the vexed problem of relapse continues to serve as a warning against any therapeutic hubris. Relapse rates remain as high in these conditions as they did before the post-war therapuetic revolution. There is argument about the prophylactic efficacy of lithium in unipolar depression, about the length of time patients who have responded to antidepressants should remain on them, about who should receive cognitive therapy and for how long.

The authors of this book are to be congratulated not merely for setting out the contemporary status of psychiatric treatment so frankly and lucidly but for placing their analysis in the context of our current knowledge concerning causality, course and outcome. They have set themselves a challenging task. The results of their exertions is a text which is relevant and sensible, erudite and accessible, topical and sound.

Preface

This book originated from case discussions in the Department of Psychological Medicine, St Bartholomew's Hospital, London. At regular meetings, patients' clinical problems are introduced by psychiatrists in training, and discussed with professionals from multidisciplinary teams in the hospital and the community. Through exposition of illness syndromes and repeated exploration of individuals' circumstance, dynamic and challenging interactions occur.

Most cases represent major health difficulties, reflecting the common existence and disabling nature of mental health problems. There is no contest to find a single treatment likely to meet patient's needs. Single modes of therapy are rarely accepted. We aim to achieve a standard of treatment through an interplay of ideas, which acknowledges that no rigid template can be applied to a given situation. Although the range of psychotropic treatments remains limited, therapy includes exploration of the origins of illness in relation to individuals' experience, and the emotive and psychological responses of the therapist.

This book is about therapy. It is not a textbook of psychiatry. We have drawn together a group of contributors to set out brief accessible accounts of a variety of common treatments. Not every treatment in psychiatry is described. Neither do we attempt to prescribe the management of specific conditions. Instead we have asked contributors to describe the essentials of the most widely applied methods in clinical practice. Most mental health workers believe in a diversity of treatments, not setting one against the other, but accepting the need for a range of methods to address patients' problems. We like Eisenberg's analogy comparing the apparently polar opposites of psychodynamic versus biological therapies to the physics of light, which has both particle and wave form. Both are essential, neither exclusive.

Gerald O'Mahony and James V. Lucey
August 1997

Acknowledgements

We wish to thank our colleagues at St Bartholomew's and at The Homerton Hospital London, the staff at John Wiley & Sons, and our contributors. We are grateful to Dr Padraig Wright, who read the text in preparation, for helpful comments.

CHAPTER 1

Treatment Planning

James V. Lucey

St Bartholomew's Hospital, London

INTRODUCTION

The treatment of mental health disorder requires co-operation and understanding. Those who share this responsibility have to consider the needs of their patients and their colleagues. No single group of remedies is entirely efficacious, and mental health therapeutics is not the exclusive domain of any one discipline. This book is intended as an introduction to a variety of treatments commonly used in psychological medicine. These treatments whether psychological or physical are typically used in combinations, often delivered by groups of professionals, working together within *multidisciplinary teams* (MDT). Management facilitates recovery, rather than cure. Ideally, patients, their families, nurses, psychologists, doctors and professionals allied to medicine, co-operate with each other and the patient; jointly enabling a return to health.

THE PATIENT, THE CLIENT AND THE ILLNESS

The treatment process begins with the patient. The term *patient* is traditionally preferred by medicine, since it implies that

Understanding Psychiatric Treatment. Edited by G. O'Mahony and J.V. Lucey.

the individual is suffering from illness and needs help. Other professional groups refer to their *clients,* stressing the co-operative, egalitarian nature, of the interaction between sufferer and carer. In practice both terms are used interchangeably.

The essential elements of mental health are the ability to live independently, to work and to love. All mental health treatment proceeds on the basis that patients or clients, have suffered significant losses of some, or all, of these capacities through psychological illness. Modern operational diagnostic systems, such as *The Diagnostic and Statistical Manual IV* (APA 1994), require that significant deterioration from previous levels of function with demonstrable impairment of well-being is present before diagnoses are made. All diagnoses in psychological medicine are *syndromes;* that is, they are collections of signs and symptoms which are recognised together. They become significant of *illness* when their distress impairs daily living. Commonly this is apparent to the patient, and *insight* is preserved. There are occasions when sufferers are not aware of their plight either through *denial,* which is an unconscious psychological defence against painful reality (Brown 1961), or through impairment of the capacity for rational thinking. In these latter situations psychiatrists may be called upon to recommend treatment without the patient's consent. This is only justified when failure to treat would result in personal ill-health or jeopardy, either to the individual or to society. Abuse of these powers led in part to the growth of the Anti-Psychiatry Movement of the 1960s, which stated erroneously that mental health disorder was a myth promoted by psychiatrists as an instrument of the state (Szasz 1962). Modern psychological medicine recognises that the origins of mental health disorder are biological, psychological and social. The manifestations are seen in all of these areas. Mental health disorders respect no boundaries.

THE THERAPEUTIC PROCESS

The basis of clinical practice is the *history,* and the most important investigation in psychological medicine is the co-lateral. This is the account by the nearest relative, or partner, or witness to the patient's suffering. The history reveals *changes* in patterns of behaviour or social interaction and accounts of personal distress. The co-lateral also reveals previous levels of functioning. One goal of treatment is to return patients to their so-called *pre-morbid state.*

The first investigation is the *mental state examination.* This reveals, among other things, the patient's attitudes, thoughts, perceptions and cognitive abilities. Morbid phenomena such as *delusions* and *hallucinations*, fears *phobias* and *rituals* may be elicited. These findings, together with the historical data, contribute to a formulation and a differential diagnosis is drawn up.

Physical, psychological and other *investigations* are proposed. Physical examination and investigation helps to out rule organic diseases which can produce psychological presentations. Infectious, inflammatory, immunological, toxic, epileptic and neoplastic processes can all present as mental health disorder. Every effort should be made to identify and exclude these treatable phenomena.

Throughout this process the patient is kept informed of the procedures. The length of time all this takes, and the setting, is dictated in part by the urgency of the problems. In the UK most mental health disorder is managed effectively in primary care general practice. Most serious mental health problems are cared for in the community and only a minority are admitted briefly to hospitals. Within the MDT a patient is usually appointed a *key worker* through whom arrangements are made to facilitate the process of history, investigation and treatment. A period of observation without specific treatment may be necessary and this may be arranged as an out-patient or an in-patient.

THE TREATMENT PLAN

Every patient is unique. An individual management plan, with review date, is essential for each patient. Its contents depend on the biological psychological and social determinants of the illness. In mental health work this *treatment plan* encompasses an understanding of the range of precipitating factors and perpetuating factors found in each client's assessment. Therapeutic strategies aimed at removing or alleviating as many of these as possible will be discussed with patients and their kin. A review date is useful since appraisal of the patient's progress is essential. Treatment plans may be modified or abandoned as the needs of the patient demand.

TREATMENTS FOR MENTAL HEALTH DISORDER

The treatments introduced in this book are all in regular use by mental health providers in the health services. Most are used in combination and the number described is not exhaustive. Physical treatments such as antidepressants, mood stabilisers, electroconvulsive therapy or antipsychotics are never used in isolation from psychological realities. Physical treatments should not be divorced from a psychotherapeutic atmosphere. Likewise psychological treatments benefit from a setting in which the biological and social contributions to illness are addressed.

Most patients make a good recovery, although, this is often forgotten. Years after the closure of the asylums, many of the fears and prejudices that hung over mental health persist anachronistically. Mental health sufferers sustain the double blow of succumbing to illnesses which limit their capacity and leave them open to *stigma* and prejudice. Now that the asylums and institutions are gone, there may be a reluctance to invest similar capital amounts into care of the mentally ill in the community. Patients who were therapeutically under-privileged in the asylums may now be physically and therapeutically under-provided in the community. There is a need for mental health advocacy on a large scale. Advocacy involves all those participating in the mental health debate, patients, relatives and the professionals. This book intends to clarify the principles underlying these shared therapeutic processes.

REFERENCES

APA (1994) *Diagnostic and Statistical Manual of Mental Disorders* (4th edition) American Psychiatric Association: Washington DC

Brown JAC (1961) The British Schools In *Freud and the Post-Freudians* Penguin Books: Harmondsworth

Szasz T (1962) In *The Myth of Mental Illness* Secker & Warburg: London

CHAPTER 2

The Place of Psychoanalytic Thinking in Modern Psychiatry

Siobhan Murphy

St Bartholomew's Hospital, London

INTRODUCTION

'In the end, Psychiatry without psychotherapy is simply dreary!' (Crisp 1996). Despite the many advances in modern psychiatric treatments, there remains a central place for psychodynamic thinking in the treatment of patients referred to psychiatrists and in the education of trainee mental health workers. Put another way, 'there is a risk that psychiatry dominated by physical methods of treatment, promoting little but physiological research related to them, will regress to unpsychological attitudes to mental disorder such as existed at the beginning of the century' (Hill 1954). This risk has changed very little in the intervening years (Pedder 1989). In the world of a sometimes bewildering expansion of 'the therapies', what is the place for a psychodynamic perspective?

Understanding Psychiatric Treatment. Edited by G. O'Mahony and J.V. Lucey.

HISTORICAL PERSPECTIVE

Modern psychoanalytic thinking is largely derived from the of the work of Sigmund Freud. His theoretical and clinical models were constantly developed and revised throughout his lifetime (Gay 1988), a process which has been continued by psychoanalysts since his death (Bateman and Holmes 1995). Major advances have been made by many psychoanalysts working in Britain, principally Anna Freud, Melanie Klein and members of their respective groups within the British Psycho-Analytical Society, as well as members of the Independent group of the British Psycho-Analytical Society, e.g. Winnicott, Fairbairn and Balint (King and Steiner 1990; Pedder 1990). Throughout these developments psychoanalysis has been concerned with three distinct areas of study:

1 The nature and role of unconscious mental processes.
2 The development of the mind and the way in which past experience influences present relationships and illness behaviours.
3 The development of the theory and clinical practice of psychoanalytic treatment (Bateman and Holmes 1995).

There are important distinctions to be made between these concepts and their potential application in psychiatry. As psychoanalytic thinking is in itself a dynamic process, a sense of the development of psychoanalytic terminology over time is useful (Sandler et al 1973; Greenberg and Mitchell 1983). Questions about the place of psychodynamic psychotherapy in modern psychiatry have tended to concentrate on the clinical practice and treatment method; whereas the use of the psychological ideas to aid thinking about the patient is sometimes forgotten. The place of analytic thinking in general psychiatry is a much broader question than a debate about the relative merits of treatment options (Holmes 1991). It includes: (1) questions about the aetiology of psychiatric disorders, about how the early environmental experiences combine with innate factors to create a predisposition to illness; (2) a way of understanding the internal world of the patient which can be used to make sense of their illness; and (3) a treatment method.

Underpinning all of these areas is the concept of the analytic attitude. This is illustrated by Main (1989) in an account of a clinical session which is also relevant to other settings in which the analyst might be working.

> The atmosphere in which the investigation is made needs consideration. It is not, despite popular belief, that of a cold analyst, tearing credulous people to pieces with painful insights.That would get nowhere, anyhow. Psychoanalysis is a collaborative effort, which eases anxieties not by processes of soothing but by understanding and interpretation of the facts behind suffering. Defences, as well as affects, are unearthed and traced to their origins in a collaborative effort. It is not a 'telling' method, as are admonition, advice, behaviour therapy, persuasion, hypnosis etc., where the therapist knows what to do. In psychoanalysis it is correctly assumed that the psychoanalyst knows nothing and has to find out. There is no consoling, no reassuring, no advice, no moralising, no judgement, no instruction, simply observation and an attempt to understand – a search for the truth. The truth itself gives trouble, because it is often painful; everyone is aware of features inside himself that he doesn't like and doesn't want other people to know about, and that he doesn't want to face honestly. The truth about unconscious features is even less welcome – they are not unconscious for nothing. The search for truth about unconscious matters can be painful and the analyst needs great care and compassion. He is aware that he will get nowhere unless this is so.

The place of formal dynamic psychotherapy in modern psychiatry is an important issue. This area and the question of the contribution of psychoanalytic thinking to the aetiology of psychiatric disorders have been recently well described (Holmes 1991; Gabbard 1994). While the treatment of the patient in formal psychotherapy is important, there are many patients for whom this might not be an appropriate treatment method but who nevertheless can benefit from being thought about in a psychodynamic way. This attempt to understand and give meaning to a patient can then be used to augment and sustain whatever treatments are being offered as well as the staff that are offering them. It might be used, for example, to understand why a patient is non-compliant with pharmacotherapy and to help him or her to maintain a medication regime.

This builds an understanding of the patient's inner world which can broaden and enrich the treatment he or she receives.

ANALYTIC THINKING AND PATIENTS REFERRED TO PSYCHIATRY

Modern psychiatry is a difficult, emotionally and physically demanding speciality which is becoming increasingly so with the move to community care and the advent of supervision registers and care programmes (Deahl and Turner 1997). Accepting their merits, these also represent an added burden to staff. With bed occupancy figures commonly over 100% in inner London hospitals (MILMIS Project Group 1995), patients spend a minimum time in hospital and often have to be discharged before staff feel they are ready. Hospital and community staff are stressed and feel overstretched, under-resourced and unappreciated. The consequences on morale and sickness rates are marked (Deahl et al 1995). In this climate psychiatrists have one of the highest suicide rates among medical practitioners. It is not only our patients who have suffered from the loss of the positive aspects of the old asylums. While they had many problems, these institutions also offered a containing function to staff as well as patients, summed up by Rey's description of them as being 'brick mothers' (see Steiner's Foreword in Magagua 1994). It is not surprising that a move away from this containment, towards poorly prepared alternative situations, has been accompanied by such distress. These more recent difficulties have added appreciably to the well-documented stresses inherent in the delivery of psychiatric services (Menzies-Lyth 1979) and their response to change (Nightingale and Scott 1994). These include the arousal in staff of painful, primitive feelings about and towards their patients stemming from complicated interactions between aspects of individual staff, individual patients and the dynamics of the institution in which they occur. The acknowledgement of these feelings and their impact on the treatment of the patient is a difficult task (Main 1989), but failure to do so increases the likelihood that the defences aroused, themselves also primitive, will become enmeshed with the treatment of the patient in a non-therapeutic way (Menzies-Lyth 1988). The acknowledgement and working through of these feelings is one of the ways that a dynamic understanding can aid the staff involved. This can be done on an individual, group or an organisational basis. Some staff will feel that their experiences with their patients has lead them towards their own therapy and one of the functions of a psychotherapist is to aid them in finding an appropriate therapist. However, a more common request is for some form of help in understanding the patient by consultation with a psychotherapist on a case work basis or by a staff support group.

The aim of the psychotherapist offering consultation to staff is to offer time and space to think about patients from a dynamic perspective; and to enable the staff members to continue working with their patients in a way which has been enhanced by understandings gained through consultation. It is not, as is often feared and sometimes hoped, to take over the care of the patient, or to decry the work already being done, by suggesting that formal psychotherapy offers the only treatment option. Part of the wider function of this work is to help staff make appropriate referrals to psychotherapy services by fostering a growing understanding of the dynamics of referring practices (Stern 1994) and other assessment issues. This work has been done either with the psychotherapist acting as consultant to a particular service (Hobbs 1990) or by offering open clinical seminars (Clark 1992) or individual consultations.

Hobbs (1990) has described a number of ways in which the psychotherapist can be asked to be involved as consultant to a psychiatric ward. These include requests to:

- conduct, or more commonly, supervise conductors of psychotherapy groups running as adjuncts to other treatments
- treat or supervise others working with selected in-patients in individual, family or specialised group therapy
- advise about the psychological aspects of management of difficult patients
- assist in the planning and development of psychological treatment programmes in the psychiatric unit
- chair community meetings, or in other ways contribute to the creation of a therapeutic milieu in the ward or unit
- support the psychiatric unit's staff, either routinely by conducting a staff support group or in other ways at times of personal or unit crisis
- contribute to the development of new models for the organisation and leadership of the team itself.

Whatever the specific request might be, Hobbs is clear that it demands an analytic stance from the psychotherapist. This depends upon the psychotherapist being sufficiently detached from the team, both administratively and clinically, to enable a psychodynamic perspective to be taken. This offers an understanding of the working of the team, and the interaction between individual, group and institutional factors. These include: the psychodynamic of the institution, the regressive effects of hospitalisation on patients, institutionalisation on staff, and the ways that individual psychopathologies can influence the functioning of a psychiatric unit.

FACTORS AFFECTING THE FUNCTION OF A PSYCHIATRIC TEAM

Example

Staff in a busy general psychiatric ward were treating a young woman with severe anorexia nervosa. Treatment was directed primarily towards weight gain as the patient was dangerously thin. Despite their best efforts, the patient failed to gain weight and anxiety about this rose steadily in the staff group. It became increasingly obvious that differences of opinion existed in the staff group about both the treatment plan and the responsibility of the patient to comply with this. Some felt that the treatment regime was too permissive, while others felt it to be draconian. The patient felt understood by these staff and miserably misunderstood by the former group. Differences of opinion were becoming increasingly apparent and were commented on by other patients. This event led to the psychotherapist being asked to provide consultation to the ward team.

Although there was some resistance to the psychotherapist being invited it was acknowledged that an impartial observer might be able to help resolve some of the difficulties which were occupying so much staff time and energy. During the period of consultation a number of factors emerged. The staff became able to discuss major differences existing in the team, about the appropriateness of treating this patient in such a unit. These feelings had not previously been openly acknowledged and were fuelled by the seeming lack of progress towards weight gain.

The meaning of gaining weight started to be discussed. Some staff were able to talk about their own confused feelings regarding eating and body size. They recognised some of the ways these had become entangled in the treatment of the patient. This led one nurse to seek help for his own previously unacknowledged eating disorder. There was also a change in the treatment to include opportunity for the patient to try to understand what weight gain might mean for her. It became obvious how the differences in the staff had led to a lack of consistency in the way she was treated, which was exploited with great ingenuity. The staff found that the process of consultation had enabled them to work with some difficult and often painful differences between themselves, helping them to present a more coherent, united, treatment plan to the patient. The patient remained a person who was difficult to treat but seemed to benefit from the more secure containment now being offered.

Some patients become 'special' and arouse very powerful emotional reactions in the staff working with them. In *The Ailment* (first published in 1957), Dr Tom Main (1989) described the splitting and projective mechanisms operating in an in-patient unit. It is as applicable to the community model more prevalent today (Obholzer 1989).

Example

A patient was referred urgently to the psychotherapy service. The letter of referral stressed the special needs of the patient and the many ways that the referring general practitioner had tried to meet these. These had some initial success but never seemed enough for the patient, whose demands escalated until it was felt that only an admission to an in-patient psychotherapy unit would be able to satisfy these needs. The doctor was exhausted, feeling that he had failed the patient. The patient had a history of profoundly disturbed early relationships, with an absent father and a psychiatrically ill mother who had been hospitalised for long periods during the patient's childhood. She had spent time in a variety of children's homes and temporary foster placements which had usually broken down.

The psychotherapist wondered if he was being asked to provide a magical solution to a lifetime of neglect, and felt this request needed further investigation before any action was taken towards in-patient psychotherapy. Enquiries revealed that there was a wide network of professionals, from mental health and social services, already involved. It was striking that most of them were either unaware of the presence of the others or, in common with the patient, rather dismissive of them. In addition to staff presently involved, there was a trail of abandoned 'others' who had vivid and negative memories of their experiences with the patient. As one said in an unguarded moment: 'Initially I thought I was really helping, but that didn't last long, – I'm not going to take her back!' A pattern of repeated referral to multiple agencies was not uncommon.

It was clear this patient aroused primitive and painful feelings in those involved in her care. Many reported a powerful feeling of needing to give this woman a different kind of relationship. The collective sense of failure in past workers was palpable, and most shared the GP's feeling of responsibility. It emerged in consultation that many had felt frightened and overburdened, often dangerously so, by the patient. They had been left feeling sucked dry, questioning their competence. These feelings had been kept secret.

In terms of help, two approaches were taken. The psychotherapist agreed to act as co-ordinator of meetings of staff presently and previously involved. These proved difficult to arrange, possibly reflecting split-off aspects of the patient; however, a degree of integration did take place, as split-up aspects of her history, and split-off aspects of her personality, were brought together and worked through. Finally a more rational, informed, care plan was developed, which took seriously the patient's considerable difficulties in making and maintaining relationships. The pattern of relationships with staff from idealisation to denigration was shared, leading to a discussion about the patient's repetition of early experiences in the present. For the staff, this was a difficult process, as many of these issues were recreated vividly within the meetings. The process offered an understanding of what was a very perplexing, emotionally charged staff–patient relationship and made a marked impact on a common sense of isolation.

The realisation of the staff's isolation, irrespective of patient–staff dynamics, led to a second approach. Many difficult psychiatric patients were being supported by inexperienced staff with limited opportunity to think about them in a coherent way. Staff felt their actions were often crisis driven, occurring without a wider understanding of the patient. This led to the establishment of open clinical seminars, run by the psychotherapist, to which staff working in general settings could bring patients for discussion. These seminars, similar to those described by Clark (1992), were based on the model developed by psychoanalysts Michael and Enid Balint in their work with social workers and general practitioners (Balint 1957). Their purpose is to provide safe, protected space and time, to think about the patient, and the way that the staff feel. Many training bodies now recognise the importance of this way of thinking about the staff–patient relationships.

The focus of these interventions is to use the feelings of staff involved with a patient to aid the understanding and treatment of the patient. Staff are unused to thinking about patients in this way and such frankness often leads to anxiety;

however, as the following example shows, this can also be, a reflection of the relationship with the patient.

Example

The psychotherapist was contacted by a member of staff who requested an urgent appointment. The departmental secretary was unusually unclear as to the purpose of the meeting, except that it was associated with a work situation. It emerged that the staff member was concerned about his feelings towards a patient who had recently told him a long-held secret about harming a child many years before. He was concerned about the effect this knowledge would have on his team and, therefore, avoided team discussions or supervision, which was quite out of character. He felt this secret should be kept, but was burdened by it.

The patient was relieved by telling someone else, but was fearful of the staff member, expecting condemnation and punitive reprisal. The staff member was flattered to have been granted this confidence, but disturbed by hateful feelings towards the patient. He felt ashamed of these intensely negative feelings.

This is a common reaction to powerful feelings aroused in staff by patients and is often kept a guilty secret. Can we hate our patients? The psychoanalyst Donald Winnicott addressed this question in his paper 'Hate in the countertransference' (Winnicott 1949). He describes reasons why a mother may understandably hate her child; and how acknowledging and understanding these powerful feelings, can help her to hold and contain her child, without acting out her feelings. A similar situation often exists between staff and their disturbed patients. Discussing the legitimacy of these feelings enabled the staff member to look at his own behaviour. He was able to see that keeping secrets from his team reflected the experience and feelings of the patient. For many years the patient felt that the knowledge was too much for anyone else to bear, and the secret was kept at great personal cost. In this situation there is a mixture of feelings: those belonging to and experienced by staff, those belonging to and experienced by patients, and those belonging to patients but experienced by staff. The consultation clarified these aspects of countertransference, transference and projective identification.

These are psychoanalytic concepts which are useful in understanding our relationships with our patients. While Breuer and Freud (1895) initially saw transference as a hindrance to treatment it has subsequently become a central tenet of psychoanalytic thinking and practice. Transference is found within all relationships and reflects the way present experience is understood on the basis of our past relationships. This includes transfer onto others of attitudes, feelings and expectations, previously experienced in important, often parental relationships. The patient above transfers the expectation of condemnation without understanding onto the staff member, expecting a pejorative response. Every relationship is a mixture of a new and a transferred relationships. Transference elements exist from the initial contact we have with our patients and probably even before. We have all had the experience of meeting someone for the first time and feeling surprised that they don't match the picture we anticipated. We have an unconscious expectation of the person, which is based on our previous experiences and affects the way we and our patients form new relationships. The awareness of transference enables us to understand the behaviour of our patients, rather than respond unthinkingly.

Example

A community nurse was allocated as the key worker for a 64-year-old woman with a long mental health history. Home visits seemed to go well, although the patient was wary and suspicious. The nurse understood that this was a new relationship in which trust would have to develop. She was perplexed to discover the patient phoning the department secretary before and after each visit, checking whether she was coming and had entered the next visit in the team diary.

The nurse had been assiduous in her attendance at visits and diary keeping. She felt her competence and professionalism were being questioned. She was tempted to raise this directly with the patient, and declare her competence. She discussed her irritation at the staff support group where she learnt that similar checks had been made on others. It was suggested this might be a transference response, reflecting the fractured relationships the patient had with her own mother and daughter. Her experience was one of abandonment, something frequently re-experienced when staff involved in her care moved on. This helped the nurse to understand and tolerate her patient's behaviour and allowed the patient to talk of her feelings about changes in staff. In this work the transference was not directly interpreted to the patient, but informed the work in the present and supported the nurse in this.

To make this kind of link there needs to be a working knowledge of the quality of the important relationships in patients' lives. It is not sufficient to have only the 'normal milestones, happy childhood' view of patients (Reiser 1988). We need to know about our patients lives and relationships, what they felt like and what this means. It is important to be able to make a psychiatric diagnosis, but this represents a starting point for understanding the patient, not an end to enquiry about the patient as an individual. All patients are unique, with their own problems, which they bring in addition to their diagnostic category.

Not all the patients' feelings towards staff are distortions. In any relationship, both parties bring aspects of themselves, past and present. The carer is as likely as the patient to have transference aspects operating. This early definition of countertransference was seen by Freud (1912) as reflecting unresolved aspects of the analyst's own conflicts and representing a barrier to analytic treatment. Even if this narrow view of countertransference is taken, it can prove useful. It enables the worker to monitor their feelings, aware that these might be more to do with themselves than with the patient.

Example

A student nurse began her placement in the day service of the local mental health unit. The treatment programme was based on group treatments into which she was invited as an observer. She was interesting and enthusiastic about the approach to the patients, with one exception. A woman of her own age was planning discharge and discussing future plans. This included the possibility of entering one of the caring professions. Staff therapists explored the meaning of this wish, and various options were discussed. In the post-group staff meeting the student expressed her irritation with the patient and the therapists. She felt that they were being indulgent of the patient, who should be told this was an inappropriate aim and directed to alternative employment. She was surprised to discover that her feelings were not shared by other staff and was perplexed by what this might mean.

The unit programme included a seminar introducing psychotherapeutic concepts to the new staff. In trying to explain the concept of countertransference, the psychotherapist invited the group to think privately about emotional responses they had towards patients. Suddenly the student made a connection between the example above and her own feelings about a younger sister, who had hero-worshipped her during her youth. While being protective towards her sister, she silently resented her wish to replicate her own actions. Her parents had not directed her sister towards alternative pursuits and the student felt she had had to struggle to have anything of her own. The feelings she experienced in the patient group were understood as belonging to her past, triggered by similar circumstances, arising with a patient who reminded her of her early experience.

This helps to understand the feelings engendered by our patients, but it does not explain the whole picture. Many patients are capable of habitually producing powerful, primitive feelings in those involved in their care that do not seem to reflect the narrow definition of countertransference given above. Countertransference is now understood in a broader way, not only reflecting the unresolved aspects of the staff, but as also something about the patient (Heimann 1950; Hinshelwood 1991; Sandler et al 1973). It has come to be seen as a powerful therapeutic tool. As the Balints said, what the doctor feels is part of his patient's illness and can be used to help understand what might otherwise seem inexplicable (Balint and Balint 1961). In this way the feelings aroused in the staff aid our understanding of the patient. Countertransference experiences involve primitive defence mechanisms of splitting and projective identification, in which the patients split off an aspect of themselves which is then projected onto the staff working with them. Gabbard (1994) describes the following situations as ones which should warn staff that processes of splitting and projective identification are occurring:

1 A staff member is uncharacteristically punitive or indulgent towards a patient.
2 A staff member repeatedly defends a patient from critical comments made by other staff.
3 A staff member believes that he or she is the only one who can understand the patient.

Projective identification is an analytic concept which provokes much debate and useful reviews may be found in Spillius (1988), Sandler (1988) and Ogden (1979). Most analysts agree that in addition to its original defensive function, in which the patient rids himself of painful states of mind (Klein 1952), it also has a communicative aspect. The patient attempts to communicate something about this painful state of mind to those involved in his care. Careful monitoring of emotional responses to patients, particularly when they seem unusual for the staff involved, can indicate the emotional world of the patient, which is not communicable more directly. Bateman (1995) describes the ways in which splitting and projective identification occur in a day hospital setting.

CONCLUSION

This chapter described some of the ways in which a psychoanalytic understanding can help staff and their patients, and enlighten apparently bizarre and meaningless behaviours. These psychoanalytic concepts throw therapeutic light on our patients' behaviours, and the interaction between them, staff members and the institutional dynamics.

REFERENCES

Balint M (1957) *The Doctor his Patient and the Illness* Pitman: London

Balint M & Balint E (1961) *Psychotherapeutic Techniques in Medicine* Tavistock: London

Bateman A (1995) The treatment of borderline patients in a day hospital setting. *Psychoanal Psychother* **9**(1): 3–16

Bateman A & Holmes J (1995) *Introduction to Psychoanalysis Contemporary Theory and Practice* Routledge: London

Breuer J & Freud S (1895) Studies in hysteria. *Standard Edition* vol 2. Hogarth Press: London

Clark A (1992) The psychotherapy clinical seminar at the Maudsley Hospital. *Psychiat Bull* **16**: 635–6

Crisp A (1996) Future directions of psychotherapy in the NHS: adaption or extinction? *Psychoanal Psychother* **10** suppl 11–20

Deahl M & Turner T (1997) General psychiatry no-man's land. *Br J Psychiat* **171**: 6–8

Deahl M Carson P & Foster T (1995) *Recognising the Limits: A Service under Siege.* Independent enquiry report to the Guys and Lewisham NHS Trust

Freud A (1936) *The Ego and the Mechanisms of Defence* Hogarth Press: London

Freud S (1912) Recommendations to physicians practising psychoanalysis. *Standard Edition* vol 12. Hogarth Press: London

Gabbard G (1994) *Psychodynamic Psychiatry in Clinical Practice The DSM-IV Edition* American Psychiatric Press: Washington DC

Gay P (1988) *Freud. A Life for Our Time* Papermac: London

Greenberg J & Mitchell SA (1983) *Object Relations in Psychoanalytic Theory* Harvard University Press: Cambridge MA

Heimann P (1950) On counter-transference. *Internat J Psycho-Anal* **31**: 81–4

Hill D (1954) Psychotherapy and the physical methods of treatment in psychiatry *J Ment Sci* **100**: 360–74

Holmes J (1991) Introduction: analytic psychotherapy In J Holmes (ed) *Textbook of Psychotherapy in Psychiatric Practice* Churchill Livingstone: Edinburgh

Hinshelwood RD (1991) *A Dictionary of Kleinian Thought* Free Association Books: London

Hobbs M (1990) The role of the psychotherapist as consultant to inpatient psychiatric units. *Psychiat Bull* **14**: 8–12

King P & Steiner R (1990) *The Freud–Klein Controversies 1941–1945* Routledge: London

Klein M (1952) Notes on some schizoid mechanisms In M Klein, P Heimann, S Isaacs & J Riviere (eds) *Developments in Psycho-Analysis* Hogarth Press: London

Magagua J (1994) *Universals of Psychoanalysis in the Treatment of Psychotic and Borderline States* Free Association Books: London

Main T (1989) The Institute and Psychoanalysis: debt differentiation and development. In T Main *The Ailment and other Psychoanalytic Essays* Free Association Books: London

MILMIS Project Group (1995) Monitoring inner London mental illness services. *Psychiat Bull* **19**(5): 276–80

Menzies-Lyth I (1979) Staff support systems: task and anti-task in adolescent institutions. In RD Hinshelwood and NP Manning (eds) *Therapeutic Communities* Routledge & Kegan Paul: London

Menzies-Lyth I (1988) *Containing Anxiety in Institutions* Free Association Books: London

Nightingale A & Scott D (1994) Problems of identity in multidisciplinary teams: the self and systems in change. *Br J Psychother* **112**: 267–78

Ogden TH (1979) On projective identification. *Internat J Psychoanal* **60**: 357–73

Obholzer A (1989) The future of psychotherapy in the NHS. *Psychiat Bull* **13**: 432–4

Pedder J (1989) How can psychotherapists influence psychiatry? *Psychoanaly Psychother* **4**(1): 43–54

Pedder JR (1990) Courses in psychotherapy: evolution and current trends. *Psychoanal Psychother* **6**(2): 203–21

Reiser MF (1988) Are psychiatric educators 'losing the mind'? *Am J Psychiat* **15**: 148–53

Sandler J, Dare C & Holder A (1973) *The Patient and the Analyst. The Basis of the Psychoanalytic Process* George Allen & Unwin: London

Sandler J (1988) *Projection Identification Projective Identification* Karnac Books: London

Spillius E (1988) Projective identification Introduction. In E Spillius (ed) *Melanie Klein Today* vol 1: *Mainly Theory* Routledge: London

Stern J (1994) The functions of a psychotherapy unit in a psychiatric hospital – refracted through the lenses of trainee psychiatrists. *Psychoanal Psychother* **8**(2): 169–83

Winnicott DW (1949) Hate in the countertransference. *Internat J Psychoanal* **30**: 69–74

CHAPTER 3

Psychotherapeutic Work in Groups

Sandra Evans and James V. Lucey

St Bartholomew's Hospital, London

INTRODUCTION

The purpose of this chapter is to clarify the role of group work as a psychotherapeutic tool, distinguishing it from one-to-one psychotherapy. Group analytic applications to areas other than formal psychotherapy will also be explored. The analysis of behaviour in groups can inform the practice of multidisciplinary teams, where it is important to consider both the effects of the institution on the individual and relationships in wider social settings.

HISTORICAL PERSPECTIVE

The importance of the group context as a therapeutic tool has been understood since the late 1930s when, in the United Kingdom, a German psychoanalyst, SH Foulkes, considered the kind of interactions his individual patients might have if they were to meet. Several years later he was given the opportunity to test out his theories at the Northfield Military

Understanding Psychiatric Treatment. Edited by G. O'Mahony and J.V. Lucey.

Hospital where, during the Second World War in parallel with Wilfred Bion and other analyst colleagues, he studied the therapeutic effects of groups on the traumatised veterans admitted there. Here, small and larger groups were conducted and observed and the beneficial effect of the 'therapeutic community' was realised (Foulkes 1948).

From their separate observations, a new set of psychodynamic theories developed which incorporated not only the analysis of the individual in the group setting but also the analysis of the group itself (Foulkes 1975). In addition, analysis by the group gave patients as group members the opportunity to interact therapeutically with each other. The group as a whole had become the subject of observation, and the group setting, the vehicle by which learning and therapeutic change took place.

Foulkesian theory was grounded in Freudian tradition which derived partly from Foulke's earlier analysis with Helene Deutsch (Foulkes 1984). This evolved further to incorporate an interpersonal understanding in addition to that of intra-psychic processing. In America a similar although not identical group therapy emerged which later resulted in a more inter-personal group and less analytic model (Yalom, 1975).

Other more structured therapeutic methods, such as psychodrama, incorporate the use of dramatic re-enactment of family and interpersonal conflicts, using role play and the subsequent debriefing of the feelings engendered (Moreno 1939).

GROUP ANALYTICAL THEORY

Object Relations Theories

The notion of working in a group setting comes from the recognition of man as a social being. Foulkes said we are 'subject to the colossal forces of society' (Pines 1983) initially from the family into which we are born and within which we develop. Human development occurs within an interpersonal setting; initially within a two-person (dyadic) mother–child relationship. Shortly afterwards three or more person relationships develop which are crucial to the group analytic concept. The school of analysis known as 'object relations theory' has influenced the group analytic understanding, particularly the work of Winnicott, Guntrip, Balint and Fairbairn.

Psychological and social development of the individual occurs within this social world, in which relatedness is considered to be essential to individual well being. A state of non-relatedness, such as autism or emotional withdrawal, is thought of as pathological. Trauma and emotional disturbance, such as separation and loss from dyadic or triadic relationships occurring during the early period of development, are of great importance in the development of subsequent emotional and mental distress (Bowlby 1980).

Treatments offered in similar settings, such as stranger groups which re-create the family unit, may be useful. Patients are given an opportunity to re-experience earlier relationships in the small group setting which confers safety and support. Foulkes preferred to call these stranger groups, proxy groups, to emphasise the transference aspect of the interaction (Foulkes 1984). Group analysis is derived from traditional psychoanalytical theory and contains all the inherent notions of unconscious process and psychological defence such as splitting, denial, projection and projective identification. Intra-psychic experiences and fantasy are worthy of consideration in group therapy, but are not given the same degree of importance they receive in an individual psychoanalysis. The patient's past experiences, memories and disappointments are aired partly for the intrinsic value of sharing them and thereby gaining relief. They also provide a context for and understanding of the patient's behaviour and responses to the group. However, if they are dwelt upon for too long, this may be a defensive measure and may block full participation in the group. The patient prefers, as it were, to relate to his or her past instead of achieving intimacy with others in the group.

Social Systems Theory

The 'Here and Now' of the patient and his or her world is brought into the group and is experienced by everyone. All members carry with them an internalised model of the world, moulded by their individual constitution and separate previous experiences. This internalised model is then projected onto the world and colours each new experience. That is, the individual behaves towards others in a way that reflects his or her expectations of them. In a small group setting, over time and with observation from all members, it becomes apparent how that internalised model concurs or conflicts with the perceptions of others.

Example

Roger, a man in his fifties, who had remembered his own father as being hypercritical, was having difficulty sustaining friendships. In the group he was intensely interested in others and would respond to them in a manner he thought was helpful. He used criteria he would apply to himself, which were perceived by the group as being harsh and judgemental. The group could now see why he was having trouble with his friends, as they were perceiving him in a similar way. This was fed back to him and he began to learn to couch his comments in a less abrasive manner. His interest in others was still appreciated and he, in turn, was shown more interest in his own story.

Example

Jane was in her early forties and had experienced enormous indifference from her mother as a small child. Her father, with whom she was close, died when she was 9 and her mother went into a depression. The consequence of her mother's bereavement was that Jane was ignored. She spent much time on her own and found difficulty in relating to others. She married a man who was as critical and detached as her mother had been, and she had great difficulty relating to her children. She had a periods of individual psychotherapy over the years, but remained desperate to feel connected to someone. She was touched by the caring assistance she received in individual therapy but found it difficult to change her perceptions of herself. In the group she repeatedly complained of feeling disconnected. In contrast, her group responded to her warmly and protested constantly that she appeared to respond to them with sincerity and interest. Jane required several years in group therapy. Over a period of time she complained less of feeling disconnected, and began to participate in her own life in a fuller and more social way.

The family, the first social system that we know, can be recreated in small group psychotherapy. *Transference relationships* that are relatively simple in individual psychotherapy, and tend to be limited to those of parental figures, can be multiple and far more complex in a group setting. Sibling rivalries are often re-enacted; intergenerational conflicts, transcultural tensions and many other types of difficult or positive social interactions may arise in the microcosmic setting of the small group.

The group analytical approach refers to a process of active and participant learning. This form of psychotherapy may be useful for individuals with a depleted sense of self, low self-esteem and who are therefore prone to depressive symptoms. *Projections* are unrecognised, unwanted aspects of an individual character, disowned and located in another individual, by psychological means. These unacceptable parts of the self may eventually be recognised, particularly if they are witnessed in other people; this is one of the phenomena referred to as the mirror reaction. These projections can theoretically be reintroduced into the *ego*, thus strengthening the sense of self. People with social and relational withdrawal, such as those with schizoid personality, may also benefit. They need time to develop trust in the other patients and in the group process to allow their defences to be broken down. Those with poor impulse control, who develop intense and potentially explosive transference attachments, respond to peer group pressure to behave and think in a more rational way. The intense transference relationships often developed by people with a borderline structure to their personality, may develop towards the group as a whole rather than be focused on one individual in particular. This diffuse transference is often safer to explore and understand under these conditions.

GROUP SPECIFIC FACTORS

In addition to psychoanalytic principles that apply in group analysis, there are a number of 'group specific' phenomena that also apply and which can be used therapeutically. These can enhance the understanding of the individual's behaviour in the group, and the group behaviour towards the individual. Such phenomena include *mirroring* which encompasses a number of different elements. It is partly about the ability to see disowned aspects of one's personality, in other group members more easily than in oneself through recognition of projection and projective defences. It is also about other group members holding a metaphorical mirror up to such individuals. This affords them the opportunity to see themselves as others see them. This can be remarkably threatening, since their deepest secret images of themselves may be negative. Time and again groups dispel these negative images by treating the disclosed terrible secret with easy acceptance or, worse, relative lack of interest. During group membership, paranoid projections of the patients are broken down and reintegrated.

Translation is the means by which symptoms become articulated and thereby conscious in the group setting. This takes time and careful consideration by the therapist and other patients. The group responds to communications occurring at a number of different levels:

1 The *here and now* level, where patients express their feelings in the group.
2 The *transference* level, where group members stand in for family members and important figures from the past.
3 The *projective* level, where patients respond to qualities in others in a positive or adverse way, but gradually learn to

recognise the similarity of their own character (Foulkes 1968).

When patients express emotions or recount personal experience, there is usually at least one group member who *resonates* to the material by expressing an evoked response in an emotional way. Such members may share their own accounts thus deepening the sense of shared intimacy, rapport and cohesiveness in the group. This may encourage people to take risks with personal material or it may enhance a sense of trust. The *matrix* refers to all of the collective experiences and communications expressed in the life of a group, which bind the individuals together in their common humanity and predicament. This web of collective experience provides a framework within which the therapeutic task can take place, and acts as a resource that grows and outlives the individual member's time in the group. The matrix has often been likened to a microbiological culture, which endures throughout the life of any one group irrespective of who comes and goes. Some essence of previous work remains, even if only in the memory of one remaining individual. Group members in slow open groups often talk of their 'ancestors', particularly when members leave or new members arrive. The matrix takes time to develop in a new group and matures over time. Mature groups seem to be able to 'contain' more effectively. They can maintain a positive therapeutic alliance and accommodate more disturbed individuals than less mature groups. As a group matures, dependency on the conductor may decrease, and patients may be more willing to challenge their therapist.

THERAPEUTIC PSYCHOTHERAPY

In psychotherapeutic models, whether group analytic or interpersonal, all the therapeutic factors of Bloch and Crouch (Nitsun 1989) come into play. The psychoanalytic and the social systems framework are in operation, making maximal use of group processes at different levels at different times.

The group setting offers additional therapeutic factors described as curative factors by Yalom (1975). These are summarised here.

1 Universality
2 Instillation of hope
3 Imparting of information
4 Altruism
5 The corrective recapitulation of the primary family group
6 Development of socialising techniques
7 Imitative behaviour
8 Interpersonal learning
9 Group cohesiveness
10 Catharsis
11 Existential factors

GROUP WORK IN HEALTH SERVICE SETTINGS

Different Applications

Different types of group work are available within the mental health sphere. These are justifiable for more than economic reasons. It may be cost effective to treat a number of people together, just as it is pragmatic to lecture a group of students together rather than teach them individually. However, students in groups also gain from each other, sharing the diverse knowledge and experience available among them.

Cognitive behavioural therapy, art therapy and some other psychotherapy models can also be conducted in groups. Hobbs (1991) offers a useful framework to think of the use of the group setting. He suggests that the group can be used as a *medium* for the performance of therapeutic activities. Any activity that can be offered on an individual basis may be included, such as exercise, ante-natal or relaxation classes, as well as anxiety management and assertiveness training.

Self-help and support groups assist in decreasing isolation and stigma associated with illness. Sharing information and help-strategies is part of the group learning process. Groups improve motivation for difficult work – for example, in dieting or resisting alcohol misuse (Weight Watchers or Alcoholics Anonymous). Other non-patient groups, such as carers' support groups (e.g. for relatives of dementia sufferers), offer support, interpersonal learning and universality which is recognition that others are in the same difficult situation as oneself. This augments the benefit of treatments or classes, and enhances a sense of community.

Example

Elsie was a depressed woman in her eighties attending a day hospital for the elderly for two years. Despite antidepressant medication, she continued to appear low in mood. She communicated little with other patients, but had a particular fondness for one member of the nursing staff. During a six-month support group employing group analytic principles, she remained silent. She revealed nothing of herself, but was patently 'in the group' in that she was alert to all that was being said. The ending of this group was painful since its members had all suffered many recent losses in their lives. Elsie finally spoke in the penultimate group. She was moved by all the stories she heard from the other patients, and expressed a felt connection with them. Elsie's husband had sustained a disabling stroke and was now taking out his anger on her. He resented her attending the day hospital, and so she felt guilty for being in the group. Now that it was coming to an end, she could appreciate the group and the others for sharing their pain and loss. Having divulged her own troubles, she felt more connected with others and they with her. She expressed a sense of decreased isolation. Elsie's persistent low mood was related to withdrawal from her own community and her guilt that she had escaped her husband's physical trauma.

Hobbs describes the group as a *milieu* or an environment, within which therapeutic change takes place. He referred to the therapeutic community, which was the analytical model at Northfield. In this setting, social and psychological therapy takes place, as people live together and learn to co-operate in a socially acceptable manner. The sense of community is enhanced by the regular community meetings, which nurture a democratic rule where the individual gives way to the needs of the community. One can see schools and the armed forces as examples of such milieu learning. Therapeutic community and ward community groups establish links between people, reducing social isolation. This provides powerful peer pressure to moderate delinquent behaviour and establishes a sense of belonging to a kind of family, often lacking in deprived individuals. Therapeutic communities exist to treat behaviourally disturbed adolescents and individuals with borderline personality. Self-harmers and people with antisocial traits can change at specialised units such as the Henderson Hospital. Research has shown this kind of unit to be effective in reducing risk of further delinquent behaviour and hospital admission (Copas et al 1996). Units such as the Cassel Hospital work with family units in distress. In the setting of family therapy (Skynner 1976), one sees an individual within the context of his or her family of origin. It tends to be most useful when family ties are strongest, at both ends of the life span, in children or adolescents and in the elderly, whose children may assume greater responsibility for them. Finally, Hobbs described the *mode* of treatment, being the small group itself. Using all the techniques described earlier, the proxy group draws on the psychoanalytical as well as the social elements in order to function therapeutically.

SMALL GROUP PSYCHOTHERAPY

The Setting

A number of factors are fixed in analytic work, including consistency of the setting, the venue the time and the therapist. A pleasant reasonably lit room, large enough to accommodate nine or ten chairs, is ideal. The optimum number of individuals in a group is eight, with equal numbers of men and women. Race and culture, age and sexual orientation of patients need to be considered in order to achieve some balance, reflection of the wider community and sensitivity to individual need.

Groups can be run as time limited treatments where all patients start and finish together, and meet on a weekly or twice weekly basis, with natural breaks. They can also be run as slow, open groups which often run for several years and patients leave as they, the conductor and the rest of the group perceive them to be ready. The length of treatment is not predetermined and depends on the change required. Long-term therapy is needed for significant changes in personality and behaviour. In the Henderson study (Copas et al 1996), for example, the optimum length of treatment was one year.

Patient Selection

Therapists, however they receive referrals, should conduct at least one assessment interview with the patient to gain an understanding of the individual's life and what the patient hopes to achieve from treatment. A willingness to reflect on one's life and an ability to look at one's behaviour critically is a requirement in all forms of talking therapies, including the cognitive behavioural treatments.

All of the criteria are open to modification. Single sex groups, for example, may be preferable for individuals who have survived sexual abuse. Foulkes (1975) suggested that heterogeneous groups worked better in the long-term treatment of personality disorder, and that a mixture of psychopathology was necessary to achieve balance. He maintained that mixing psychopathology and character strengths allowed an exchange of qualities across members, thus achieving a normalisation of the individual.

Most people who fulfil the criteria required for selection in individual psychodynamic therapy are also treatable in groups. The requirement that individuals are *psychologically minded* is universal. Contra-indications to group work are few. Destructive or violent people would be too threatening. Paranoid individuals may become more alienated, and mind-

or mood-altering drugs or alcohol are strongly discouraged as they interfere with the ability to communicate and to remember. This does not preclude patients from taking prescribed anxiolytics or antidepressant medication which may help them to concentrate and be more psychologically available for the therapeutic task.

Group Breaks and Endings

Natural breaks are an important factor in any dynamic therapeutic relationship. Losses and endings may resonate with patients who respond in an unconscious fashion, often called 'acting out'. This may involve coming late to sessions or not coming at all for several weeks. The message can be interpreted as 'If you abandon me, then I don't need you'. It is important to be aware of the negative consequences of breaks, holidays and endings, including staff changes. Patients in hospital for weeks or months develop strong attachments to staff members and need preparation for parting and time to say goodbye.

NEGATIVE ASPECTS OF GROUPS

Negative aspects of groups include mass hysteria and the abdication of individual responsibility such as the unthinking behaviour experienced in football crowds. Foulkes' own experience of Nazi Germany is another example. The negative and feared aspects of group work can be explored in order to understand ourselves more fully as individuals, and as members of society. This understanding may harness potential therapeutic energy and avoids pitfalls when working with vulnerable groups.

The first principle to consider is adequate training and supervision in group work. Multidisciplinary team members need training and support when called upon to run community groups (Sharpe 1995). Experienced observers will note that the most manic patient typically sits in the centre of the circle and takes up all available space, demonstrating how groups amplify and expose psychopathology. Groups by their nature elicit anxiety, particularly large groups. There are tensions between feeling that one might be rejected or attacked by the group, and conversely fearing being overwhelmed by the group, losing one's sense of self and individuality. Both these fears are examples of primitive and paranoid fears of annihilation. Nitsun (1991) proposes the term *antigroup* as an umbrella term for destructive forces that attack the therapeutic process or which threaten the integrity of the group itself.

It is a difficult and time-consuming task to start up and run a stranger group. People often have a fear of groups and express a preference for individual work. Initially, the conductor or therapist is seen as the holder of the key to health. Others are seen as potential obstacles to the conductor, and at one level that is the reality. There is only the one therapist and seven or eight individuals who might see themselves as rivals rather than the fellow travellers that Foulkes envisaged. As in Yalom's (1975) Rabbinical vision of Heaven and Hell – where Heaven was only distinguished by the co-operation of its inhabitants – patients can help each other to restore their own psychological well-being. Conversely with individuals who cannot co-operate with each other and who distrust themselves, therapeutic work may be made impossible and group destruction becomes inevitable.

There is a tension in wanting to be in the group enjoying a sense of community, and fearing the groups threat of loss of individuality. The entire group then meets with anxiety and ambivalent feelings. It may be that ambivalence and healthy scepticism are required for therapeutic interventions to occur, but too much absence by members conveys worthlessness to those who remain, particularly if their sense of self worth is tenuous.

Angry and destructive feelings in a group may be misdirected or expressed in identifying a *scapegoat* – a group member who becomes the repository for all that is wrong with the group. The group might share the fantasy that, if the scapegoat were to be expelled, all would be right with the world. It is imperative that the conductor identifies scapegoating if it arises both to protect the individual from a potentially damaging experience; but also to protect the group from its own destructiveness. When people leave groups because of difficult circumstances, they leave behind a sense of loss and failure, from which a group might never recover.

Owing to selection errors, unsuitable individuals may enter groups. These people may be full of scorn for others and treat the group with contempt. They may challenge the conductor and invite retaliation. They may be incapable of self-reflection or progress, becoming increasingly alienated from the group. It is often kinder to remove these individuals and find them a more appropriate form of treatment. They should always be offered something as the experience of being rejected from a group is a difficult one and needs to be worked through, particularly if one wishes to learn from the experience and to avoid repetition. A patient who is disruptive in a group and who invites rejection may be recreating an earlier rejection, hence the need for the therapist to know of the patient's previous history and remain alert to this possibility.

Example 4

In a case of double mirror reaction, or malignant mirroring (Zinkin 1983), two men found themselves embroiled in bitter exchanges. Jeff had embraced contemporary gay culture as expressed in his style of dress and uncompromising language. Tom had not had a relationship with anyone, man or woman and found Jeff's accounts of his exploits intolerable and judged him harshly. Jeff in return found Tom sanctimonious and told him so. The resulting arguments took up a great deal of group time and threatened the therapeutic work of the group. Only the therapist who had seen both men individually before entering them into the group knew that both harboured a private anxiety about their sexuality. They appeared to have unconsciously recognised that in each other, but were unable to deal with the discomfort it brought to themselves. The therapist needed to work with them actively or require one to leave to prevent them from adversely affecting the group.

RESEARCH AND EFFICACY STUDIES

Yalom suggested it is unrealistic to expect research to effect great change in our practice. Unlike the case in physical medicine, many aspects of what psychotherapists do are difficult to quantify, particularly those interactions which are subjective and unique to each individual therapist. It may be a strength of psychotherapy that, despite the lack of 'concrete' evidence, it has a strong culture and following in the Western world. Pressures on health services resources are increasing the demand for accountability. Born out of this is the call for 'evidence-based medicine' which is a challenge increasingly being met.

Data are difficult to compare since group therapy differs across studies and between centres. Comparisons between group-treated patients and non-group-treated controls invariably show greater improvements in those participating in groups – this is despite the fact that significant improvements can also be seen in untreated patients (Piper et al 1977). Studies of group therapy show clear early benefits for depressed adolescents in groups which addressed self-esteem and cognitive distortion, compared to groups which simply provided social skills training (Fine et al 1991). However no differences were apparent at nine months follow-up. In substance-dependent men, increasing the duration of participation in group psychotherapeutic programmes, as part of aftercare, improves outcome and recovery significantly (Lash and Dillard 1996). Longer term benefits were shown in group therapy, which included conjoint marital work for recovering alcoholics, compared to standard individual therapy. Conjointly treated patients had significantly lower alcohol consumption at six months follow-up. The trend was also apparent at one year. The couple element within their group therapy facilitated greater maintenance of recovery (Bowers and Al Redha 1990).

Group-based psychotherapy can have psychodynamic, cognitive or behavioural content. When the effect on outcome of interpretation in psychodynamic and behavioural group psychotherapy was examined, the greatest improvements were seen when behaviour patterns were interpreted. Most therapists, whether analytical or behavioural, interpreted present behaviour rather than the distant past (Flowers and Booraem 1990). In one long-term follow-up study of analytical group psychotherapy (Malan et al 1976) there was a strong positive correlation between favourable outcome and previous individual psychotherapy. Nonetheless, the authors questioned the value of switching patients from individual therapy to group analytical approaches (Malan et al 1976). There is more positive experience within therapeutic communities. In a study of 48 residents, the majority of whom had borderline personality disorder, significant symptom reduction was demonstrated at three and six months. Clients rated group therapy as the most helpful component of the program (Hafner and Holme 1996).

WIDER APPLICATIONS OF GROUP ANALYTIC THEORY

Group analysis can have a wider role in the context of organisations. Mental health workers rarely work alone. The role of an individual in a multidisciplinary team has potential problems as well as benefits. We may learn more about ourselves within different group settings such as committees or larger organisations. Organisations are not only theoretical structures that rely on members knowing their place and role; they are also closed systems, in which changes in one area will affect others. As institutions grow in size, there is an equivalent need for the sustained growth of communication channels. Problems arise when communication breaks down and the potential rises for primitive anxieties such as paranoia (Main 1957). It is useful here to extrapolate to larger groups some of the small group dynamics explored above. Tasks of the organisation, in the health services, of treating patients, reducing distress and cutting costs, may put individuals in difficult or stressful situations. Mechanisms to cope with such stresses may be satisfactory, such as good lines of communication and support from managers, or they may be misdirected causing fractures between managers and clinical staff, and putting pressures on both sides. All who work in health services should be aware of the work of Isobel Menzies-Lyth (1959), who described a clinical setting in which the management of the task was being carried out to the emotional detriment of staff and patients alike.

CONCLUSIONS

Humans exist in societies; that is our setting. We define ourselves by our family of origin, our culture, our era or generation and the work and social groups into which we invest our time and energy. Illness and distress, born out of loss of attachment to groups or people, associated with difficulties in relating to and communicating with others, can be usefully treated in group settings. An understanding of how groups work or malfunction is a skill that can enrich and inform most areas of our clinical work.

REFERENCES

Bloch S, Crouch E & Reibstein J (1981) Therapeutic factors in group psychotherapy. *Archives of General Psychiatry* **38**: 519

Bowers TG & Al Redha MR (1990) A comparison of outcome with group/marital and standard/individual therapies for alcoholics. *J Alcohol Stud* **51**: 301–9.

Bowlby J (1980) *Attachment and Loss* vol 3. *Sadness and Depression* Penguin Books: Harmondsworth. Reprinted 1991. First published Hogarth Press 1980

Copas J, O'Brien M, Roberts J et al (1996) Treatment outcome in personality disorder. The effect of social, psychological and behavioural variables. In B Dolan (ed) *Perspectives on Henderson Hospital* Henderson Hospital 1996

Fine S, Forth A, Gilbert M & Haley G (1991) Group therapy for adolescents with depressive disorder: a comparison with social skills and therapeutic support. *J Am Acad Child Adol Psychiat* **30**: 79–85

Flowers JV & Booream CD (1990) The frequency and effect on outcome of different types of interpretation in psychodynamic and behavioural group psychotherapy. *Internat J Group Psychother* **40**: 203–14

Foulkes ET (1984) The origins and development of group analysis. In TE Lear (ed) *Spheres of Group Analysis* GAS Publications

Foulkes SH (1948) *Introduction to Group Analytic Psychotherapy* Heinemann: London. Reprinted 1983 with permission by H. Karnac Books

Foulkes SH (1975) *Group Analytic Psychotherapy, Methods and Principles.* First published 1975. Reprinted Maresfield Library 1991

Hafner RJ & Holme G (1996) The influence of the therapeutic community on psychiatric disorder. *J Clin Psychiat* **52**: 461–8

Hobbs M (1991) Group processes in psychiatry. In J Holmes (ed) *Textbook of Psychotherapy in Psychiatric Practice* Churchill Livingstone, Edinburgh

Main TF (1957) *The ailment. Br J Med Psychol* **30**: 129–45

Malan DH, Balfour FH, Hood VG & Shooter AM (1976) Group psychotherapy. A long term follow-up study. *Arch Gen Psychiat* **33**: 1303–15

Moreno JL (1939) Psychodramatic shock therapy. *Sociometry* **2**: 1–30

Menzies-Lyth I (1959) The functioning of social systems as a defence against anxiety. *Human Relations* **13**: 95–121

Nitsun M (1989) Early development: linking the individual and the group. *Group Anal* **22**: 249–60

Nitsun M (1991) The anti group: destructive forces in the group and their therapeutic potential. *Group Anal* **24**(1): 7–20

Pines M (1983) The contributions of SH Foulkes to group-analytic psychotherapy. In M Pines (ed) *The Evolution of Group Analysis* International library of group psychotherapy and group process. Routledge & Kegan Paul: London

Piper WE, Debane EG & Garant J (1977) The outcome of group therapy. *Arch Gen Psychiat* **34**: 1027–32

Sharpe M (ed) *The Third Eye. Supervision of Analytic Group Psychotherapy* Routledge: London

Skynner ACR (1976) *Systems of Family and Marital Psychotherapy* Brunner/Mazel: New York (British Edition): *One Flesh: Separate Persons* Constable: London

Yalom ID (1975) *Theory and Practice of Group Psychotherapy* (2nd edn) Basic Books: New York

Zinkin L (1983) Malignant mirroring. *Group Anal* **16**(2): 113–25

CHAPTER 4

Social and Community Psychiatry

Kamaldeep Bhui and Dinesh Bhugra

Institute of Psychiatry, London

INTRODUCTION

The term 'social and community psychiatry' evades precise definition. 'It is concerned with the effects of the social environment on the mental health of the individual, and with the effects of the mentally ill person on his or her social environment' (Leff 1993). Another more detailed definition states that

> Social psychiatry is concerned with the contextual factors and forces which affect human development, especially aberrant development, culminating in mental ill health, including adverse environmental conditions, such as poverty or famine, as they relate to the incidence and prevalence of mental illness. Therefore social psychiatry focuses on relationships beginning with intra-uterine life, as well as on macro-social conditions as they influence personal development, family, groups, and communities regarding health or illness. Furthermore, social psychiatry is associated with treatment contexts in the institutions and the community, as well as the incidence and distribution of mental illness in a given population. (Fleck 1990)

Understanding Psychiatric Treatment. Edited by G. O'Mahony and J.V. Lucey.

Areas of concern shared by mental health and sociology include: the family and socialization, homelessness, employment and leisure, education and religion; urbanization, social policy and the distribution of wealth; criminality and deviance, race and social class. In this chapter, we will consider social support, homelessness, unemployment, social class and the family, briefly discussing them in relation to community psychiatry as the clinical arm of social psychiatry.

HISTORY AND DEVELOPMENT

'Social psychiatry' as a term was first used to bridge the gap between the mental hygiene movement and the new profession of social work in 1917 (Cooper 1995). Social psychiatry developed as a branch of scientific medicine. As individuals, we are a social species, recruiting novel, creative and abstract methods of communication. Through these we maintain a relatedness to each other and our environment. Occasionally distortions arise in our social selves and in our communications. Such distortions are the subject matter of psychiatry. Psychiatrists rely on 'conversation samples' to discover the patients' internal world and unspoken states of being, as well as their relatedness to themselves, their peer group and society. Eisenberg (1995) suggests that all psychiatry is both biological and social: 'There is no mental function without social context. The cyto-architecture of the cerebral cortex is sculpted by input from the social environment, because socialization shapes essential human attributes in our species.'

CONTROVERSIES WITHIN SOCIAL PSYCHIATRY

Cooper (1995) outlines the hostility to which social psychiatry has been subjected; these attacks are worrying as they arise from professionals who were formerly advocates. Sartorius (1988) writes that 'Social Psychiatry will disappear and this world would be a better place without it'. Jablensky (1990) challenged the assumption that social psychiatry is a concrete entity with specified component structures and tasks. Accordingly he wrote that conceptual changes were inevitable. Whether social psychiatry survives or not is irrelevant, since the continuing social fabric of psychiatry is not in doubt (Jablensky 1990). Social psychiatry is not a label; it is a process. The process is of psychiatry trying to relate to and serve society, in the real world and time frame in which our patients experience ill health. To study mental illness devoid of social context, produces a schism between the social reality of mental illness and the interpretation of the sufferer's experience (Thomas, Somme and Hamelijnck 1996). This repression of our social selves in psychiatric practice explains some of the criticisms of psychiatrists by our clients (Rogers, Pilgrim and Lacey 1993).

Cooper (1995) asserts that social psychiatry has a number of potential flaws.

> Its philosophy may extend beyond its remit into social engineering and political reform. It is divisive, since it assumes the existence of an opposite pole to non-social psychiatry. It has reinforced the tendency to pursue social and biological research separately, instead of developing unifying theories. So far it has failed to identify effective preventive measures.

Different parties locate themselves in the social sphere of psychiatric practice. Their emergence leads to conflicts of professional identity (Leff 1993). Thus psychotherapists, epidemiologists, transcultural psychiatrists, life-events researchers, students of expressed emotion and health service researchers, can all be placed within social psychiatry.

Social psychiatry's polar relationship to biological science could arise from the emphasis given to biological formulations of health and illness. Patients desire non-medical solutions wherever possible. Recent attention to homelessness (Bhugra 1993a), HIV (King 1993), race and culture (Leff 1988; Bhugra 1993b) come from psychiatrists aware of political and economic contexts. Purely biologically orientated psychiatrists may question the value of these considerations, when the scientific approach is focused on pharmacological treatment. This does not adequately address those affected with disability, or acknowledge that changing social realities can have a therapeutic effect. The task of socially aware mental health professionals is to synthesize the bio-medical research and clinical agenda. Biological research needs to incorporate social psychiatry and shift the attention of professionals to environmental and relationship issues.

The influence of social factors on healthcare was increasingly recognized in the 1970s and 1980s (Scrivens and Holland 1983; Fox and Adelstein 1978). Psychiatry discovered its social variables through serendipity rather than planned study. Tooth and Brook (1961) prematurely reported that the long-stay asylum population was declining such that it would be eliminated within 16 years. Weller (1993) recently exposed these predictions as ill-founded. Such announcements were resonant with the civil liberties movement in psychiatry. The asylums built for 'pauper lunatics' in the UK reached their largest capacity in 1954 when there were 151 400 residents (Weller 1993). The hospital plan for England and Wales proposed the closure of these hospitals regardless of the unexplained variation in beds across the country. Goffman (1961) was at that time developing social models of mental disorder. Predominant biological or degeneracy theories were replaced by labelling theory and interpretations of mental illness as social deviance. Reorganization of psychiatric institutions influenced the physical and mental well-being of patients (Wing and Freudenberg 1961), and social environmental effects influencing the well-being of patients with schizophrenia were studied (Wing and Brown 1970).

COMMUNITY PSYCHIATRY AS THE NEW SOCIAL PSYCHIATRY

Epidemiology is the scientific arm of social psychiatry; community care is its clinical arm (Fleck 1990). Social psychiatry is psychiatry free from the institutions and located on the high street, in the patient's familiar surroundings. Large converted houses, providing 24-hour care for the mentally ill, may appear as satellite asylums, evoking much public concern (Brockington et al 1993; Wolff et al 1996). Community psychiatry will have failed if it effects nothing more than shifting the locus of care (Thomas, Somme and Hamelijnck 1996) without addressing areas shared between mental health and sociology. Knowledge of the therapeutic community (Jones 1953), instrumental family environments (Brown et al 1972), and the ideological implications of de-institutionalization (Wing and Furlong 1986) can each contribute. Social psychiatrists believe that without addressing prejudice and stigma from communities as well as professionals, opportunities for change will have been lost.

The principles of community psychiatry have been outlined recently by Bennet and Morris (1993). They state that:

- the environment of people with mental health disorder should be the same as that of the community and that segregation from society is not acceptable
- changing the locus of community care as a panacea is also unacceptable
- an active approach is necessary to maximize the function of the severely mentally ill
- medical and hospital services are components of community care; they are not alternatives to it.

COMMUNITY CARE

In recent years community based approaches to mental health services have become encumbered with ideological concerns obscuring the reality of service provision (Falloon and Fadden 1993). De-institutionalization invoked high expectations of patients, the public and professionals. Such moves require both the discharge of patients from long stay hospital wards, and the development of sustained resources for quality community care. Hospital care affords respite to families, watching their relatives deteriorating in chronic illnesses. Neither processes of institutionalization nor de-institutionalization were carried out on a basis of systematic research; rather on the political will and ideology of the time. Notwithstanding studies indicating that home care is no worse than hospital care (Hoult 1986; Muijen et al 1992; Onyett, 1990), ill informed optimism has led to the re-creation of the same deprivation found in the institutions. The reformers' enthusiasm was tempered by the realization that serious mental disorder is not cured by human warmth and understanding (Lamb and Goertzel 1970). A co-ordinated strategy is necessary if community care provision is to reach those with mental health needs.

Service goals should be set so that resources are allocated efficiently (Falloon and Fadden 1993). A community care system based on sectorization should include the following components (Strathdee and Thornicroft 1993):

1 Crisis response and acute care
2 Continuing care and outreach
3 Consultation and liaison
4 Day care
5 Respite
6 Attention to physical health
7 Housing
8 Family and community education and support
9 Rehabilitation and resettlement services.
10 Peer support.

CASE MANAGEMENT

Different models emphasise adaptation of the ideology of community care to specific populations (Lavender and Holloway 1991; Muijen 1993). Case management is one by which services can be co-ordinated. It encompasses co-ordination, integration and allocation of individualized care within limited resources (Thornicroft 1991). The principles of case management are:

1 Accessible services
2 Needs assessment
3 Continuity of care
4 Fostering independence
5 Patient advocacy
6 Advocacy for services
7 Therapeutic staff–patient relationships.

The core tasks of case management include case finding, ensuring access to the service, designing a care package, and coordinating service delivery. The care plan should be modified through review evaluating effectiveness of services. The implementation of case management programmes should reflect local need.

Social Support and Models of Care

A stress vulnerability model has been proposed, whereby illness arises from a combination of inherent and environmental factors, which overcome the individuals bio-psycho-social adjustment (Falloon and Fadden 1993). Vulnerability predisposes an individual to a disorder at a given time. Rehabilitation encourages patients to work on their deficits and build on their strengths. The advent of the therapeutic community in the post-war era is a good example of the way social psychiatry developed. The therapeutic community is dependent upon interpersonal relationships between the staff and patients and between patients themselves. The emphasis is on social functioning. This is a normalizing process. Purposeful activity is at the core of the therapeutic community helped by social work involvement and planned rehabilitation.

A modification of the therapeutic community model gave rise to *Milieu Therapy*, which is broadly similar to rehabilitation therapy and aims to increase skills and encourages adaptive social behaviour. These approaches involve the manipulation of the social environment to the advantage of the patient.

Social Class

Social class serves as a indicator of adverse environments. The links between social class and psychiatric morbidity and the validity of hypothesized mechanisms are debated. Faris and Dunham (1939) demonstrated that patients with schizophrenia were found in areas of Chicago that were subject to social disorganization; these include poor inner cities with a high profile of drug and alcohol misuse. Goldberg and Morrison (1963) alternatively hypothesized this arose because of social drift, so that illness led to social decline. The 'breeder hypothesis' of Faris and Dunham (1939), that people living in inner cities are truly more likely to develop schizophrenia, has been recently revisited (Lewis et al 1992; Dauncey et al 1993). Early environments including in-utero states and obstetric complications, maternal influenza and childhood head traumas are all possible causal links (Buszewicz and Phelan 1994).

Great attention is now directed to the inner city and the characteristics of urban environments of aetiological significance. Brown and Harris (1970) demonstrated that a confidant was of value in the prevention of depression among working-class women in Camberwell, and that having two children under the age of 14, and being at home jobless with these children, were vulnerability factors. Social class is known to be associated with marriage, divorce and single parenthood (Argyle and Henderson 1985) and is important as a risk factor in its own right. The highest divorce rates are for social class III (non-manual) and class V (unskilled workers). Middle-class divorces occur later in life when a more mature personality may be able to cope with adversity and isolation. Less-educated couples encounter more physical and psychological abuse. Suicide rates in cities were previously higher than in rural areas, but in recent years this trend has reversed and especially so for men. Compared with the general population, those who commit suicide are more likely to have been divorced, unemployed, or to be living alone in social isolation (Sainsbury 1955).

Homelessness

The closure of the institutions was thought responsible for the increased visibility of the mentally ill among homeless populations (Lamb 1984). Two-thirds of the homeless mentally ill in London suffer from schizophrenia. Nearly 90% of the seriously mentally ill become homeless after their first episode of illness; loss of accommodation is a direct result of their mental illness. Hidden homeless categories include those who squat or stay on relatives' floors or occupy hospital beds. Lelliot, Sims and Wing (1994) identified that between 25 and 50% of acute psychiatric admission beds were occupied by homeless people. In one inner London study nearly 60% of residents in homeless women's hostels had previously been admitted to psychiatric hospitals. The majority were suffering from schizophrenia. Less than half of those diagnosed as schizophrenic were in contact with mental health services (Marshall and Reed 1992). Similar high rates of psychiatric morbidity were seen in a community-based study in the USA. The homeless with a previous history of psychiatric hospitalization were least likely to avail of emergency shelters, were homeless nearly twice as long, and had the worst mental health status. They used more alcohol and drugs and were more involved in criminal activity (Gelberg, Linn and Leake 1988).

Abrahamson (1993) outlined the process of setting up rehousing schemes for the severely mentally ill. A range of accessible accommodation is necessary, from independent living to high support residential group homes. Thompson (1994) outlined the consensus on the necessary admixture of different levels of supported accommodation. The need is for 40 to 150 staffed 24-hour residential places for a population of 250 000; 30 to 120 day staffed places and 50 to 125 acute psychiatric care beds. Any community care strategy must account for the homeless population, otherwise scarce resources from the acute services will be used to support failing social provision.

THE FAMILY

In studies of family relationships and mental health disorder the concept of expressed emotion (EE) has been influential.

Using audio-taped family interviews, symptoms and coping responses were observed. Sources of irritation, and the use of time in a typical week, were used as the basis of ratings of relationship characteristics. Critical comments, hostility, emotional over-involvement, positive remarks, and warmth were the core EE phenomena identified; the first three are the most predictive. Schizophrenic patients in families with low EE have relapse rates (21%) less than half that of high EE groups (48%). Kavanagh (1992) and Bebbington and Kuipers (1994) carried out a meta-analysis of the world literature and confirmed that EE was strongly predictive of relapse. Carers and staff interactions with patients could either precipitate relapse or perpetuate illness. Interventions to reduce EE environments were either preventative of relapse or reduced relapse rates to levels seen in low EE environments. Thus the subjective burden on the patient is lightened and social performance and family atmosphere are improved (Kuipers 1995).

Education alone has not proved to be of benefit, although relatives' groups have reduced EE and improved social performance. Kuipers (1992) indicated that those relatives living with patients who relapse more than once per year, despite compliance with treatment, frequently contact staff for help and reassurance. Kuipers (1992) prioritizes those requiring EE work: families in which there are repeated arguments with verbal or physical violence, any family that calls the police, and single relatives, usually mothers, looking after the patient without assistance. Training workers to deliver social interventions to families with a severely mentally ill relative is at an early stage.

UNEMPLOYMENT

Work provides structure and financial stability in peoples lives, allowing the individual to be occupied usefully, contributing to society's growth and economy. It also enhances self-esteem, effective relationships with colleagues, exposes workers to interpersonal and hierarchical relationships, and gives some experience of dealing with conflict, forming social networks and gaining support.

Employment is an institutionalized social relationship, with mutual contractual obligations. The relationship of unemployment and psychological morbidity was studied (Jahoda, Lazarsfeld and Zeisel 1933/1972) when the impact of factory closure in an Austrian village was observed. Many of the community were dejected, resigned and hopeless. Depression following unemployment is well recognized.

The psychological effects of unemployment include debilitation, economic insecurity, exhaustion, poor self-esteem and despondency (Bakke 1940). A strong ecological relationship exists between parasuicide and completed suicide and levels of socio-economic deprivation including unemployment (Gunnell et al 1995). Unemployment explained 50 to 60% of the variance in admission rates in different areas of Bristol in a two-year study (Kammerling and O'Connor 1993). Thornicroft, Margolius and Jones (1992) found that 55% of the variance in new long-stay psychiatric admissions were related to measures of socioeconomic deprivation on the Jarman Index in four London districts and 81% were associated with local rates of unemployment. Unemployment may be a chronic difficulty contributing to depression. Major psychosocial transitions, akin to life events, are changes occurring over a short time span with lasting effects on the individual's assumed world (Murray-Parkes 1971). Mental health professionals need to recognize the impact of unemployment and related poverty as precipitating and perpetuating psychiatric morbidity. The impact of unemployment on groups like women, youth, and ethnic minorities needs acknowledgement and further study.

URBANIZATION

The advance of urbanization, with its associated social dislocation, may contribute to changing patterns of mental health disorder; with a profound impact on the delivery of services. Through a concentration of effects on those at highest risk, resource problems increase, requiring planning for appropriate responses to meet these needs. For example, the report assessing *London's Mental Health* (Kings Fund 1997) records that London is at the extreme of the national spectrum of unemployment (16.5%) compared to the national average (9.2%). The capital has the six districts in England with the highest levels of social deprivation: 36% of its population is aged 15 to 45 years, compared to 29% nationally – the years most associated with risk for mental health disorder; there are more single-person households (54% versus 27% nationally); it has the highest proportion of ethnic minorities (77% of the UK's black Africans and 58% of black Caribbeans); it has more homeless with 50% of the nation's rough sleepers; and has the majority of refugees. Substance misuse rates are the highest of the UK. Seventy per cent of AIDS cases notified annually are found in London (Kings Fund 1997).

CULTURE, SOCIAL POLICY AND ANTI-PSYCHIATRY

Cultural awareness is essential in psychiatry practised in a multicultural society (Kleinman 1977). Psychiatry should consider the influence of oppression, socio-economic discrimination and racism on mental health. Taken to extremes, this social awareness led to the untenable proposal by the *Anti-psychiatry Movement* of the 1960s that there was no physical causation for mental illness, and that it was society which was 'sick' rather than the individual (Szasz 1962; Laing 1960). Certainly the interaction between the individual and society is potentially an oppressive one. In response, social psychiatry has affected social policy; for example, studies of institutionalization were influential in encouraging psychiatry and political leaders to move towards treatment in the community (Wing and Brown 1970).

Epidemiological data are needed to help clinicians develop services (Mann 1993). Solutions for mental illness derived from epidemiological research might require government initiatives rather than clinical activity. This is in keeping with social theories of mental illnesses, and the social psychiatrist's goal in promoting greater public acceptance of the mentally ill (Mann 1993). Community epidemiological studies suggest that psychiatric disorder, especially minor psychological morbidity, is more frequent in society than previously thought. This may reflect better diagnosis or a genuine increase in morbidity due to urbanization, changing social and family structures, or other social factors described above.

A study of the contribution of socio-economic risk factors to the incidence and maintenance of psychiatric disorder in primary care (Weich et al 1997) found that a high prevalence of disorders reflects chronicity rather than an unduly high incidence. Risk factors associated with onset differed from those associated with maintenance of psychiatric disorder. Clinical risk factors may have their greatest effect on the onset, while socio-economic risk factors contribute to the prevalence of disorders by prolonging existing episodes.

CONCLUSION

Multidisciplinary mental health professionals attempt to provide a *bio-psycho-social* assessment and a management plan, recognizing the social contributions to ill health and the ways in which its treatment must be mediated by social understanding.

REFERENCES

Abrahamson D (1993) Housing and deinstitutionalisation. In M Weller & M Muijen (eds) *Dimensions of Community Care* Saunders: London

Argyle M & Henderson M (1985) In *The Anatomy of Relationships* Penguin: London

Bakke WW (1940) In *Citizens Without Work* Yale University Press: New Haven, CT

Bebbington P & Kuipers E (1994) The predictive utility of expressed emotion in schizophrenia: an aggregated analysis. *Psychol Med* **24**: 707–18

Bennet D & Morris I (1983) Deinstitutionalisation in the United Kingdom. *Internat J Ment Health* **11**(4): 5–23

Bhugra D (1993a) Unemployment, poverty and homelessness. In D Bhugra and J Leff (eds) *Principles of Social Psychiatry* Blackwell: Oxford

Bhugra D (1993b) Influence of culture on presentation and management of patients. In D Bhugra & J Leff (eds) *Principles of Social Psychiatry* Blackwell Scientific: Oxford

Brockington I, Hall P, Levings J & Murphy C (1993) The communities tolerance of the mentally ill. *Br J Psychiat* **162**: 93–9

Brown G & Harris T (1970) In *Social Origins of Depression* Tavistock: London

Brown G, Birley J & Wing J (1972) Influence of family life on the course of schizophrenic disorders: a replication. *Br J Psychiat* **121**: 241–58

Buszewicz M & Phelan M (1994) Schizophrenia and the environment. *Br J Hosp Med* **42**(4): 149.

Cooper B (1995) Do we still need social psychiatry? *Psychiatrica Fennica* **26**: 9–20

Dauncey K, Giggs J, Baker K & Harrison G (1993) Schizophrenia in Nottingham: lifelong residential mobility of a cohort. *Br J Psychiat* **163**: 613–19

Eisenberg L (1995) The social construction of the human brain. *Am J Psychiat* **152**: 1163–75.

Falloon I & Fadden G (1993) *Integrated Mental Health Care* Cambridge: Cambridge University Press

Faris R & Dunham H (1939) *Mental Disorders in Urban Areas* University of Chicago Press: Chicago

Fleck S (1990) Social psychiatry – an overview *Social Psychiat & Psychiat Epidemiol* **25**: 48–55

Fox A & Adelstein A (1978) Occupational mortality: work or way of life? *J Epidemiol Comm Health* **32**(2): 73–8

Gelberg L, Linn LS & Leake BD (1988) Mental health alcohol and drug use and criminal history amongst homeless adults. *Am J Psychiat* **145**: 191–6

Goffman, I (1961) *Asylums: Essays on the Social Situation of Mental Patients and Other Inmates* New York: Anchor Books

Goldberg E & Morrison S (1963) Schizophrenia and social class. *Br J Psychiat* **109**: 785–802

Gunnell DJ, Perters TJ, Kammerling RM et al (1995) Relation between parasuicide, suicide, psychiatric admission and socioeconomic deprivation. *Br Med J* **311**: 226–30

Hoult J (1986) Community care of the acutely mentally ill. *Br J Psychiat* **149**: 137–44

Jablensky A (1990) Public health aspects of social psychiatry. In D Goldbert & D Tamtam (eds) *Public Health and Social Psychiatry* Hogrefe & Huber: Toronto

Jahoda M, Lazarsfeld P & Zeisel H (1933/1972) *Marienthal: The Social Sociography of an Unemployed Community* Aldine-Athenton: New York

Jones M (1952) *Social Psychiatry* Tavistock: London

Kammerling RM & O'Connor S (1993) Unemployment as predictor of rate of psychiatric admission. *Br M J* **307**: 1536–9.

Kavanagh D (1992) Recent developments in expressed emotion and schizophrenia. *Br J Psychiat* **160**: 601–20

King M (1993) Psychological and social aspects of AIDS. In D Bhugra & J Leff (eds) *Principles of Social Psychiatry* Blackwell: Oxford

Kings Fund (1997) *London's Mental Health* Kings Fund vol 1, pp 4, 5

Kleinman A (1977) Depression, somatisation and the 'new cross-cultural psychiatry': *Soc Sci Med* **11**: 3–10

Kuipers L (1992) Expressed emotion in Europe. *Br J Clin Psychol* **31**: 84–94

Kuipers L (1995) EE assessment, intervention and training. In T Brugha (ed) *Social Support and Psychiatric Disorder* Cambridge University Press: Cambridge

Laing R (1960) *The Divided Self* Tavistock: London

Lamb U (1984) De-institutionalization and the homeless mentally ill. *Hosp Comm Psychiat* **35**: 889–907

Lamb H & Goertzel V (1970) Discharged mental patients – are they really in the community? *Arch Gen Psychiat* **24**: 29–34

Lavender A & Holloway F (1991) Models of continuing care. In M Birchwood & N Tarrier (eds) *Innovations in Psychological Management of Schizophrenia* John Wiley: Chichester

Leff J (1993) Principles of social psychiatry. In D Bhugra & J Leff (eds) *Principles of Social Psychiatry* Blackwell: Oxford

Lelliot P, Sims A & Wing J (1994) Who pays for community care? The same old question. *Br Med J* **307**: 991–4

Lewis G, David A, Andreasan S & Allebeck P (1992) Schizophrenia and city life. *Lancet* **340**: 137–40

Mann A (1993) Epidemiology. In D Bhugra & J Leff (eds) *Principles of Social Psychiatry* Blackwell: Oxford

Marshall EJ & Read J (1992) Psychiatric morbidity in homeless women. *Br J Psychiat* **161**: 761–7

Muijen M, Marks I et al (1992) Home based care and standard hospital care for patients with severe mental illness: a randomized controlled trial. *Br Med J* **304**: 749–54

Muijen M (1993) Mental health services: what works? In M Weller & M Muijen *Dimensions of Community Care* Saunders: London

Murray-Parkes C (1971) Psychosocial transitions: a field for study. *Soc Sci Med* **11**: 101–15

Onyett S (1990) The early intervention service: the first 18 months of an Inner London demonstration project. *Psychiat Bull* **14**: 267–89

Rogers A, Pilgrim D & Lacey R (1993) In *Experiencing Psychiatry: Users' Views of Services* MacMillan: London

Sainsbury P (1955) Suicide in London. The epidemiology of suicide. In A Roy (ed) *Suicide* Williams & Wilkins: Baltimore

Sartorius N (1988) Future directions: A global view. In Henderson PS, Burrows GD (eds) *Handbook of Social Psychiatry*. Elsevier: Amsterdam, pp 341–6

Scrivens E & Holland W (1983) *Inequalities in health in Britain. A critique of the report of a research working party. Prev Health Care* **1**(2): 97–103

Strathdee G & Thornicroft G (1993) The principles of setting up mental health services in the community. In D Bhugra & J Leff (eds) *Principles of Social Psychiatry* Blackwell: Oxford

Szasz T (1962) In *The Myth of Mental Illness* Secker & Warburg: London

Thomas P, Somme M & Hamelijnck J (1996) Psychiatry and the politics of the underclass. *Br J Psychiat* **169**: 401–4

Thompson K (1994) *Housing and Serious Mental Illness. A review of the research on the link between housing and mental health.* Report to the Department of Health

Thornicroft G (1991) The concept of case management for long term mental illness. *Internat Rev Psychiat* **3**: 125–32

Thornicroft G, Margolius O, Jones D (1992) The TAPS project 6. New long stay: Psychiatric patients and social deprivation. *Br J Psychiat* **161**: 621–4

Tooth G & Brook E (1961) Trends in mental hospital populations and their effect on future planning. *Lancet* **1**: 710–13

Weller M (1993) Where we came from: recent history of community provision. In *Dimensions of Community Mental Health Care* Saunders: London

Weich S, Churchill R, Lewis G & Mann A (1997) Do socioeconomic risk factors predict the incidence and maintenance of psychiatric disorder in primary care? *Psychol Med* **27**: 73–80

Wing J & Furlong R (1986) A haven for the severely disabled within the context of comprehensive psychiatric community services. *BrJ Psychiat* **149**: 449–57

Wing J & Freudenberg R (1961) The response of severely ill chronic schizophrenic patients to social stimulation. *Am J Psychiat* **118**: 311–22

Wing J & Brown G (1970) *Institutionalism and Schizophrenia* Cambridge University Press: Cambridge

Wolff G, Pathare S, Craig T & Leff J (1996) Community attitudes to mental illness. *Br J Psychiat* **168**: 183–90

CHAPTER 5

Physical Treatments for Depression

Timothy G. Dinan

Department of Psychiatry, Royal College of Surgeons in Ireland, Dublin

INTRODUCTION

Major depression is one of the commonest of all medical conditions with a lifetime prevalence of 4% (Weissman et al 1988). The risk of developing depressive disorder increases with age and females are at a higher risk than males. Psycho-social stress, early development and genetic factors all play a part in determining risk (Paykel 1982).

Considerable progress has taken place in recent years in terms of the operational definition of psychiatric illnesses. The evolution of such operational definitions has been of considerable help in a clinical setting and also in drug development. The Diagnostic and Statistical Manual (DSM-IV) criteria for diagnosing major depression are listed in Table 5.1 and have a high inter-rater agreement (APA 1994). Patients with major depression can be further categorised into those with melancholic symptoms, such as early morning wakening and weight loss, or psychotic symptoms which should be mood congruent. All recent studies of antidepressants have made

Understanding Psychiatric Treatment. Edited by G. O'Mahony and J.V. Lucey.

Table 5.1 Criteria for major depressive episode

A. Five (or more) of the following symptoms have been present during the same two-week period and represent a change from previous functioning; at least one of the symptoms is either (1) depressed mood or (2) loss of interest or pleasure.
   (1) depressed mood most of the day, nearly every day, as indicated by either subjective report (e.g. feels sad or empty) or observation made by others (e.g. appears tearful)
   (2) markedly diminished interest or pleasure in all, or almost all, activities most of the day, nearly every day (as indicated by either subjective account or observation made by others)
   (3) significant weight loss when not dieting or weight gain (e.g. a change of more than 5% of body weight in a month) or decrease or increase in appetite nearly every day
   (4) insomnia or hypersomnia nearly every day
   (5) psychomotor agitation or retardation nearly every day (observable by others, not merely subjective feelings of restlessness or being slowed down)
   (6) fatigue or loss of energy nearly every day
   (7) feelings of worthlessness or excessive or inappropriate guilt (which may be delusional) nearly every day (not merely self-reproach or guilt about being sick)
   (8) diminished ability to think or concentrate, or indecisiveness, nearly every day (either by subjective account or as observed by others)
   (9) recurrent thoughts of death (not just fear of dying), recurrent suicidal ideation without a specific plan, or a suicide attempt or a specific plan for committing suicide.

B. The symptoms do not meet criteria for a Mixed Episode.

C. The symptoms cause clinically significant distress or impairment in social, occupational, or other important areas of functioning.

D. The symptoms are not due to the direct physiological effects of a substance or a general medical condition.

use of the DSM operational criteria. The effectiveness of antidepressants in sub syndromal cases, which do not fulfil the criteria (and are commonly seen in primary care) is debatable.

HISTORY AND DEVELOPMENT

Prior to the 1950s no effective pharmacological treatments were available for managing depression (Leonard and Spencer 1990). The 1950s saw a major breakthrough in the development not only of antidepressants but also in the development of anti-schizophrenia drugs. In the middle of that decade, the first monoamine oxidase inhibitors (MAOIs) were synthesised. The development was largely based on the fortuitous observation that anti-tuberculous drugs with an MAOI structure produced an elevation in mood. The MAOIs phenelzine, tranylcypromine and iproniazid were rapidly marketed. Within a short period of time, the first tricyclic antidepressants, imipramine and amitriptyline, became available (Kuhn 1958). These two categories of antidepressant have remained a cornerstone in the pharmacological management of depression until relatively recently.

In the 1970s and 1980s a number of novel antidepressants were developed but showed a variable market penetration. The most notable of these drugs are mianserin, nomifensine and trazodone (Richelson 1987). They have a mechanism of action considerably different from the MAOIs or the tricyclics. Trazodone established itself as an antidepressant in the US but made considerably less impact in the UK. Mianserin, on the other hand, was used by some clinicians in Europe for the treatment of depression in the elderly, especially where insomnia was a problem, but the drug was never marketed in the US. Nomifensine was withdrawn shortly after launch because of unforeseen adverse events.

VARIOUS DRUGS AND THEIR USES

The development of the selective serotonin re-uptake inhibitors (SSRIs) represents the most important pharmacological breakthrough in antidepressant therapy since the 1950s. The notable members of this class are fluoxetine, fluvoxamine, sertraline, paroxetine and citalopram (Feighner and Boyer

1991). A similar development of note is that of venlafaxine, described pharmacologically as a selective serotonin and noradrenaline re-uptake inhibitor (SNRI) (Dinan and Burnett 1997). Moclobemide is another recent development belonging to the MAOI category. The uses and mechanisms of action of these various drugs will be described briefly.

Tricyclic antidepressants (TCAs)

There are now numerous TCAs available which include imipramine, amitriptyline, desipramine, dothiepin, clomipramine and trimipramine. These drugs act at central synapses by blocking the re-uptake of serotonin and/or noradrenaline (see Figure 5.1). Some drugs are more potent in inhibiting the re-uptake of noradrenaline, for example desipramine, while other drugs have a more potent action at the serotonin synapse, for instance clomipramine. These observations gave rise to Schildkraut's catecholamine hypothesis of depression (Schildkraut 1965). As a category of drug they are highly effect as antidepressants but are especially toxic in overdose and have significant side-effects. Their side-effects profile relates to the fact that they block a variety of receptors, including cholinergic and noradrenergic receptors. Common unwanted side-effects include dry mouth, blurring of vision, constipation and sedation. In higher doses, these drugs do affect the heart and can be especially cardiotoxic in the elderly.

Commonly prescribed doses of TCA's are often considerably below effective doses. For most healthy adults, amitriptyline and related drugs should be prescribed in excess of 150 mg per day for therapeutic efficacy. In primary care the majority of patients receive considerably less than this. A major disadvantage of these drugs is the fact that the starting dose must be considerably lower than the therapeutic dose. Most patients commence on 50–75 mg daily and escalate in steps over a 1–3 week period. As suicide is always a risk in the management of depression, such agents are especially hazardous. One week's prescription of amitriptyline, if taken in

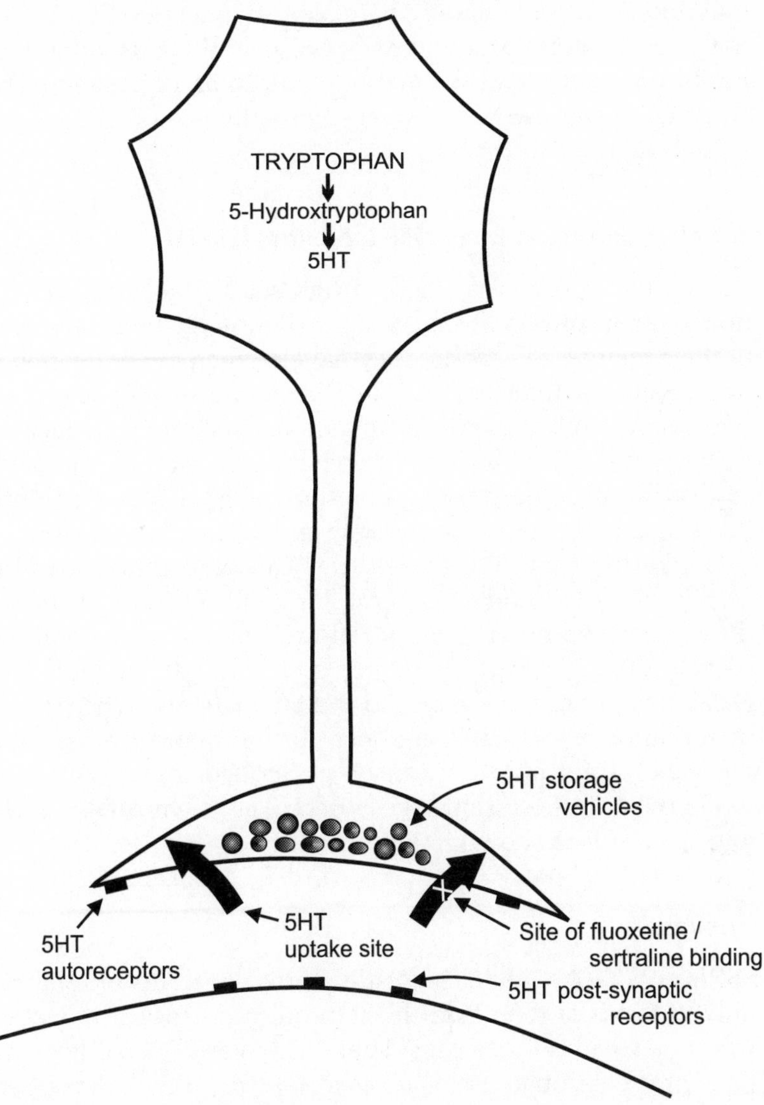

Figure 5.1 Structure of the serotonin synapse showing the site for active uptake of serotonin, which is blocked by antidepressants. The impact of such a block is to acutely increase the concentration of serotonin in the synapse

overdose, can prove fatal. The major advantage of TCAs lies not only in terms of low cost but also in their usefulness in promoting sleep and alleviating symptoms of anxiety. The chemical structures of the most commonly used TCAs can be seen in Figure 5.2.

Selective Serotonin Re-uptake Inhibitors (SSRIs)

As the name suggests, these drugs act by blocking the re-uptake of serotonin at the synapse (Baumann 1992). Because of their relative selectivity, they have a much lower incidence of side-effects than the tricylics. In overdose they are relatively safe, do not impair psychomotor performance such as driving, and do not have the anticholinergic side-effects, such as dry mouth. The most troublesome side-effects seen with these agents are nausea, headache and sexual dysfunction.

Unlike the tricyclics, these drugs can be commenced at a therapeutic dose and in general are well tolerated at such a dose. The therapeutic dose for fluoxetine and paroxetine is usually 20 mg per day and for sertraline 50 mg per day. Escalation of dosage is required in some patients. Where sleep disturbance is a major component of the depression, a benzodiazepine for sedation can be prescribed for a short time while the antidepressant takes effect. The chemical structure of some SSRIs is shown in Figure 5.3.

Comment

SSRIs and TCAs cannot be distinguished in terms of efficacy, only in terms of their side-effects profile and cost. If the latter was not an important consideration it would be difficult to justify the continued use of TCAs for the majority of depressed patients. Given the burden of side-effects caused by TCAs, a strong economic argument can be put forward to justify the use of SSRIs, despite their increased cost. Furthermore, over the past three years the cost of SSRIs has fallen sharply.

Apart from their use in the treatment of depression, these drugs have also been demonstrated to be effective in the

Tertiary Amines

Secondary Amines

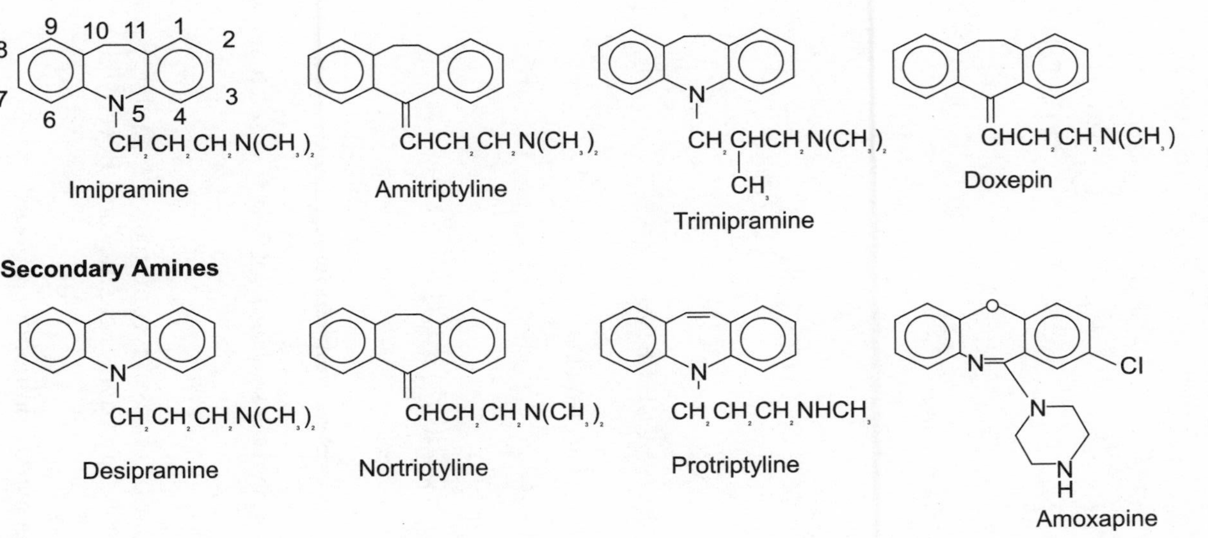

Figure 5.2 Chemical structures of most commonly used tricyclic antidepressants

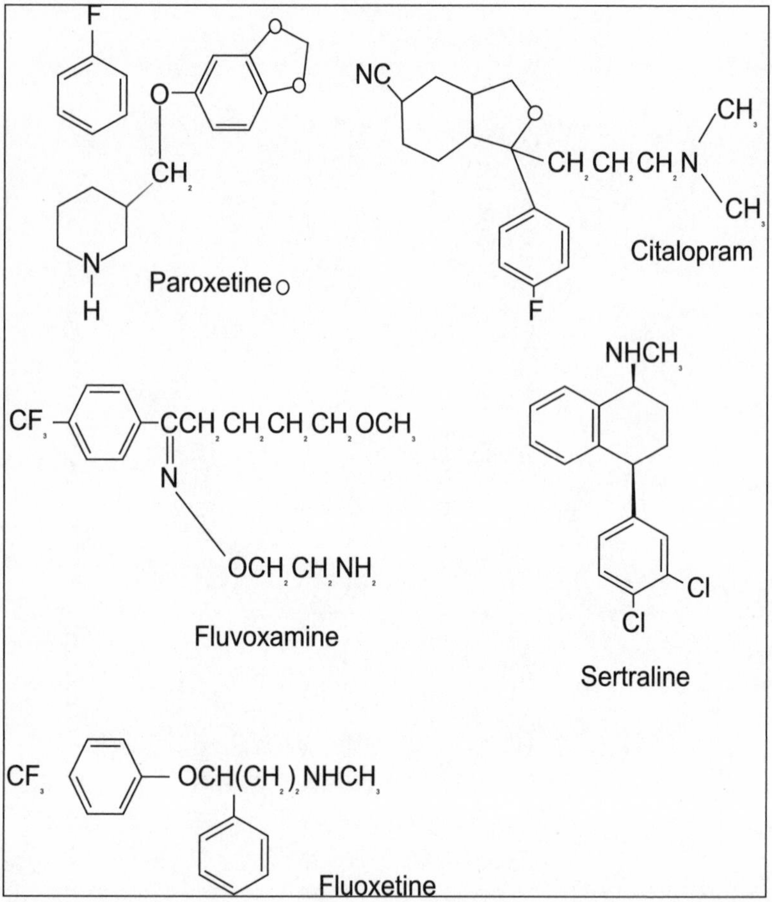

Figure 5.3 Chemical structures of selective serotonin re-uptake inhibitors

management of obsessive compulsive disorder, panic disorder and eating disorders (Feighner and Boyer 1991).

Monoamine oxidase inhibitors (MAOIs)

There are two types of MAO enzyme, A and B, and both of these are inhibited by traditional MAOIs. Because of potential interactions with various foods and with a variety of drugs, the MAOIs are now only occasionally prescribed. Potentially dangerous increases in blood pressure occur when tyramine-containing foods are ingested in the presence of MAOIs. Cheese, some red wines and alcohol-free lagers are especially high in tyramine and should be omitted from the diet when taking an MAOI. Despite these obvious limitations, there are occasions when MAOIs can be especially beneficial.

Patients with an atypical depression profile have been shown to benefit from MAOIs (Pare 1985). Atypical depression is characterised by a depression of mild to moderate severity, a high level of anxiety, perhaps with agoraphobia and an inverse physiological shift in the form of hypersomnia and hyperphagia. Phenelzine is the most widely used MAOI and is usually commenced at 15 mg three times a day. This is an adequate therapeutic dose in some patients, but others require considerably higher doses. The major determinant is the acetylator status of the patient. Those patients who are slow acetylators require low doses, while higher doses are required in rapid acetylators.

Moclobemide is a reversible inhibitor of MAO-A and is, therefore, considerably safer. The dietary restrictions required with the old drugs are not required with moclobemide. Theoretically, the impact of older drugs is achieved by inhibition of MAO-A. Whether the selective moclobemide is as effective as its older counterparts is the subject of clinical debate. However, several placebo-controlled studies have demonstrated it to be an effective antidepressant.

Other Recent Drugs

Venlafaxine is an SNRI which is well tolerated and is claimed to have a broader spectrum of action than the SSRIs (Dinan and Burnett 1997). It has also been suggested that it may have a more rapid onset of therapeutic action, but the evidence for this is less clear-cut. It is generally commenced in doses of 37.5 mg twice daily and escalated as required. Overall, it is an effective drug which is well tolerated.

Nefazodone is a weak blocker of serotonin uptake and also blocks serotonin receptors. It is a sedative drug which is useful in promoting sleep. Its efficacy in the management of milder forms of depression is beyond doubt. Whether it is as effective in severe forms of depression is debatable. Mirtazapine is another antidepressant with a dual mode of action blocking as it does noradrenergic alpha-2 receptors and serotonin 5-HT2 receptors. As it is relatively new to the market, experience with it to date is limited. Nonetheless, it does show promise (Kasper 1995).

RATIONALE FOR ANTIDEPRESSANT USE

The monoamine hypothesis of depression has held sway for over a quarter of a century. This proposes that depression is due to a reduction of serotonin and/or noradrenaline in certain central synapses (Coppen and Doogan 1988). Recent efforts to modify the hypothesis have suggested that the abnormality lies not in the concentrations of neurotransmitters but in the sensitivity of the receptors at which they act. For example, rather than a decrease in the synaptic concentration of serotonin, it may be that the serotonin receptor post-synaptically is less sensitive. Antidepressants act by acutely increasing the concentrations of neurotransmitter within the synapse and, over a two- to four-week period, increasing the sensitivity of the post-synaptic receptor. Clinical response most accurately is reflected by a change in the sensitivity of the post-synaptic receptor.

The major limitation of this monoamine hypothesis is that no attempt is made to link the biology of depression with the most obvious observation that depression occurs in a setting of stress or negative life events. Recently, Dinan (1994) has attempted to link the social literature on depression with the above biological hypothesis, by assuming that the overwhelming majority of depressive episodes occur in a setting of life stresses. In such a setting, the individual exhibits a series of psychological and biological responses. The core stress response in man, at a biological level, is activation of the hypothalamic-pituitary-adrenal (HPA) axis. When this system is activated, cortisol levels rise rapidly. Cortisol is a steroid produced by the adrenal gland, which is of major importance in adapting to stress. Most patients with severe depression show elevations in their cortisol levels. Unlike healthy subjects, who also increase cortisol in response to stress, depressives elevate their cortisol but show an inability to switch off the response. Depression can therefore be conceptualised as a sustained stress response. Inappropriate cognitive strategies may bring about the maladaptive stress response.

It is now well recognised that cortisol has a powerful impact on the brain (De Kloet and Reul 1987). Cortisol influences the brain through two types of receptor. The type 1 receptor (mineralocorticoid receptor) is found in the septo-hippocampal projection, while the type 2 receptor (glucocorticoid receptor) is found throughout the brain and in especially high concentrations on those serotonin and noradrenaline neurones. Dinan (1995) proposes that the alterations in serotonin and noradrenaline seen in depression are brought about by the very high levels of cortisol induced as part of the stress response.

This model, while helping to explain the action of antidepressants, incorporates a psychosocial component which recognises the importance of psychological strategies in the management of depression. Figure 5.4 outlines the model.

TREATMENT RESISTANCE

At best, antidepressants are effective in about 70% of patients and, on average, take two to three weeks to produce a response (Dinan 1995). Before any patients are described as treatment resistant, it should be demonstrated that they have taken an adequate dose and an adequate duration of treatment. The minimum duration required before making this decision is at least six weeks. Treatment resistance may result

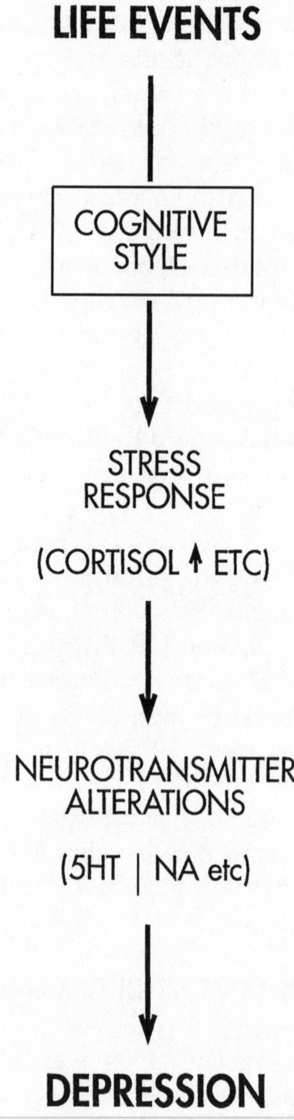

Figure 5.4 A psycho-biological model of depression. The impact of stress on cortisol is shown, together with the subsequent changes in noradrenaline (NA) and serotonin (5HT). The fact that cognitive structuring influences the biological response to stress is emphasised

from ongoing psychosocial stress or comorbid physical illness such as thyroid disease (even when treated), occult carcinomas, previous minor head injuries or heavy alcohol consumption which may counteract the antidepressant.

Many combinations of medications have been used in the treatment of resistant patients but the addition of lithium to the antidepressant is undoubtedly the most extensively investigated strategy (De Montigny, Gonberg and Mayer 1981). Lithium is known to augment the actions of TCAs and SSRIs. In general, the combination is effective and side-effects largely relate to an exacerbation of the side-effects caused by the antidepressant on its own. There is a theoretical risk of developing a severe condition called the serotonin syndrome. This is potentially life threatening but is extremely rare.

Electroconvulsive therapy (ECT) is an important treatment for both severe and resistant cases of depression. Originally developed in 1938 by Cerletti, the Italian psychiatrist, it has remained an important treatment for depression. Especially in the elderly, where severe forms of depression can be associated with rapid dehydration and profound anorexia, ECT can be life saving. Several studies have now demonstrated its efficacy beyond doubt. The Medical Research Council (1965) sponsored a multi-centre random allocation study involving 269 patients who were treated either with ECT, imipramine, phenelzine, or placebo. The response rate in the ECT group was in excess of 70% while the response rates in the other groups were as follows: imipramine 53%, phenelzine 30%, placebo 39%. More recently, the Northwick Park study compared real ECT with simulated ECT (Johnstone, Lawler and Stevens 1980). With simulated ECT the patients simply received an anaesthetic but no convulsion was induced. The short-term outcome in the ECT-treated group was better than that in the simulated ECT group. Several other studies have reported similar findings.

While the need for ECT is clearly decreasing as better pharmacological treatments become available, ECT is nonetheless, a powerful tool in the management of severe forms of depression.

PSYCHOTIC DEPRESSION

This is a relative rare and severe form of depression, characterized by core depressive symptoms and mood-congruent delusions and hallucinations. Psychotic features often relate to worthlessness, poverty, sinfulness or hypochondriacal ideas. These episodes do not usually respond to monotherapy. A combination of an antidepressant and an antipsychotic is required. ECT is also highly effective.

MAINTENANCE THERAPY

Following an acute episode of major depression, antidepressants should be maintained for at least six months. Given the relapsing nature of depression, some patients may require long-term prophylaxis. The dose of drug used for maintenance should be the same as that used to treat the acute episode. Previously it was thought that maintenance could be achieved at a dose below that required for treating the acute episode. This is not the case, the dose that results in recovery is the dose necessary to keep the patient well.

Patients are often reluctant to continue with antidepressants once they have recovered. In practice over 50% of patients relapse in a nine-month period if antidepressants are withdrawn following the acute episode (Doogan and Caillard 1992). That continuation of the antidepressant will reduce the risk is now beyond doubt.

OTHER PHYSICAL TREATMENTS

Light therapy in the form of high-intensity artificial light (2500–10 000 lux for up to 2 hours is given in the mornings) has been advocated, especially for those patients with depressive episodes prone to occur in the winter (Blehar and Rosenthal 1989). Despite enthusiasm for such a strategy in the popular press it remains largely experimental in use. A similar strategy, perhaps worth considering in resistant cases, is sleep deprivation. A temporary alleviation of symptoms may be achieved with deprivation in the second half of the night. The combined use of sleep deprivation and lithium shows promise (Baxter et al 1986).

Psychosurgery remains an effective treatment for severe intractable depression. It is now used only in the most resistant of cases and it can produce remarkable benefit. For patients to be considered for surgery their symptoms should be severe, be unresponsive to ECT, present for more than two years, failed adequate doses of different antidepressants and psychotherapeutic and social interventions (Bridges and Bartlett 1977). Strict stereotaxic procedures are followed, unlike the free-hand surgery of former times. The bi-frontal subcaudate tractotómy is one of the more common procedures and involves the planting of radioactive yttrium seeds. Recovery rates of around 60% are reported and improvement is not seen for four months after surgery.

CONCLUSIONS

The past 40 years have seen major advances in the treatment of depression. Significant breakthroughs took place in the 1950s with the development of TCAs and MAOIs. Over the past decades, newer preparations have emerged with a far lower incidence of side-effect and a relative safety in overdose. The major challenge for the future is the development of antidepressants which work more rapidly and are effective in more than 70% of patients.

REFERENCES

APA (1994) *Diagnostic and Statistical Manual of Mental Disorders* (4th edition) American Psychiatric Association: Washington

Baumann P (1992) Clinical pharmacokinetics of citalopram and other selective serotonergic reuptake inhibitors (SSRIs) *Internat Clin Psychopharmacol* **6** (suppl 5): 13–20

Baxter LR, Liston EH, Schwartz JM et al (1986) Prolongation of the antidepressant response to partial sleep deprivation by lithium *Psychiat Res* 1917–23

Blehar MC & Rosenthal NE (1989) Seasonal affective disorders and phototherapy: report of a National Institute of Mental Health-sponsored workshop *Arch Gen Psychiat* **46**: 469–74

Bridges PK & Bartlett JR (1977) Psychosurgery yesterday and today *Br J Psychiat* **131**: 249–56

Coppen AJ & Doogan DP (1988) Serotonin and its place in the pathogenesis of depression *J Clin Psychiat* **49**: 4–11

DeKloet ER & Reul JMH (1987) Feedback action and tonic influence of corticosteroids on brain function: a concept arising from the heterogeneity of brain receptor systems *Psychoneuroendocrinol* **12**: 83–105

De Montigny C, Gonberg S & Mayer A (1981) Lithium induces rapid relief of depression in tricyclic antidepressant non-responders *Br J Psychiat* **138**: 252–6

Dinan TG (1994) The role of steroids in the genesis of depression: a psychobiological perspective *Br J Psychiat* **164**: 365–72

Dinan TG (1995) Treatment approaches to therapy-resistant depression *J Psychopharmacol* **9**: 199–204

Dinan TG & Burnett F (1997) Venlafaxine: pharmachology clinical efficacy and tolerability of a serotonin–noradrenaline reuptake inhibitor. *J Serotonin Res* **3**: 161–75

Doogan DP & Caillard V (1992) Sertraline in the prevention of depression. *Br J Psychiat* **160**: 217–22

Feighner JP & Boyer WF (eds) (1991) *Selective Serotonin Reuptake Inhibitors* Wiley: Chichester

Johnstone EC, Lawler P & Stevens M (1980) The Northwick Park electroconvulsive therapy trial *Lancet* **2**: 137–45

Kasper S (1995) Clinical efficacy of mirtazapine: a review of meta-analyses of pooled data. *Internat Clin Psychopharmacol* **10** (suppl 4): 25–35

Kuhn H (1958) The treatment of depressive states with G22355 (imipramine hydrochloride). *Am J Psychiat* **115**: 459–64

Leonard B & Spencer P (eds) (1990) *Antidepressants: Thirty Years On* CNS: London

Medical Research Council (1965) Clinical trial of the treatment of depressive illness *Br Med J* **ii**: 881–6

Pare CMB (1985) The present status of monoamine oxidase inhibitors *Br J Psychiat* **146**: 576–84

Paykel ES (1982) Life events and early environment. In ES Paykel (ed) *Handbook of Affective Disorders* Guilford: New York, pp 146–61

Richelson E (1987) Pharmacology of antidepressants *Psychopathol* **20** (suppl 1): 1–12

Schildkraut JJ (1965) The catecholamine hypothesis of affective disorders: a review of supporting evidence *Am J Psychiat* **122**: 509–22

Weissman MM, Leaf PJ, Tischler GL et al (1988) Affective disorders in five United States communities *Psychol Med* **18**: 141–53

CHAPTER 6

Behavioural and Cognitive Treatments

Anne-Marie O'Dwyer

Maudsley Hospital, London

INTRODUCTION

The last 40 years have seen the development of effective behavioural treatments for a variety of psychiatric disorders. This chapter will trace the evolution of behaviour therapy and its theory, as this provides an understanding of the rationale for many behavioural interventions. It will then outline the elements of a behavioural approach, focusing primarily on anxiety disorders. The development of cognitive therapy will be discussed. The final section will review evidence for the efficacy of behavioural interventions. It is hoped that this chapter will provide the reader with an understanding of how behaviour therapy developed, what a programme of behaviour therapy entails for a patient, what patients are likely to benefit from behavioural treatment and where cognitive therapy fits in a behavioural approach to psychiatric disorders.

Understanding Psychiatric Treatment. Edited by G. O'Mahony and J.V. Lucey.

BEHAVIOUR THERAPY: A HISTORICAL PERSPECTIVE

Evolution of Behaviour Therapy: Origins and Theory

The term 'behaviour therapy' (BT) was first used about 40 years ago. The origins of behaviour therapy can be traced back to models of animal learning and behaviour, based largely on the work of Pavlov and Skinner. Pavlov described a form of animal learning termed *classical conditioning* – repeated pairing of an unconditioned stimulus with another stimulus (conditioned stimulus) leads to the conditioned stimulus alone eliciting the original response. Pavlov also demonstrated that this process could be 'unlearned' – repeated presentation of the conditioned stimulus without the unconditioned stimulus led to gradual disappearance of the conditioned response (a process termed *extinction*). While limitations of the classical conditioning model of human fears and phobias are now recognised (Davey 1992), Pavlov's work provided the cornerstone for the development and application of behavioural principles to anxiety disorders. Another model of conditional learning, *operant conditioning*, was developed by Skinner and his colleagues. This was based on earlier work by Thorndike, Tolman and Guthrie, who found that behaviour consistently followed by satisfying consequences is repeated, while behaviour followed by unpleasant consequences occurs less frequently. Skinner developed this principle further – defining *positive reinforcement* (increase in behaviour because of reward) and *negative reinforcement* (increase in behaviour due to omission of an anticipated aversive event). *Aversive conditioning* (behaviour followed by an unpleasant event) and *frustrative non-reward* (behaviour not followed by anticipated reward) both led to reduction in the relevant behaviour.

These two models of animal learning came, largely, to be associated with two distinct fields of development of behaviour therapy – Skinnerian principles adopted largely by American researchers, and Pavlovian ideas by British researchers. American behaviour therapy was practised largely by psychologists who were radically committed to a behavioural understanding of all mental disorders, concentrating exclusively on behaviour. The Skinnerian model was applied to severely ill, institutionalised patients with chronic, often intractable problems such as schizophrenia, mental handicap and self-harming behaviour. 'Token economy systems' were developed for severe, psychotic, behavioural disturbance and, later, for patients with learning disability (Ayllon and Azrin 1968).

The British approach remained distinct from the American one. Psychiatrists as well as psychologists contributed to the field; an acceptance of genetic influence and a more eclectic approach to mental illness was evident. The British concentrated largely on neurotic disorders – in particular anxiety disorders. Anxiety disorders, particularly phobias, were considered to be manifestations of conditioned fear with conditioned responses evidence by avoidance behaviours. Mowrer (1960) incorporated both classical and operant conditioning theories in his explanation of fear and avoidance behaviours. He proposed a two-stage model to account for fear and avoidance behaviour. Fear of stimuli is acquired through classical conditioning. The animal then learns to avoid conditioned stimuli to reduce fear. Any avoidant or other behaviour that reduces anxiety will thus be reinforced. Developments in conditioning theory suggest that the conditioning theory of fear acquisition is not a sufficient explanation (Rachman 1991). Nonetheless, it provided the basis for behavioural treatment of anxiety disorders, in particular phobias.

Applications of Behavioural Techniques

Watson and Rayner's description of conditioning of fear in 'Albert' provided the basis for much of the early development of behavioural treatments (Watson and Rayner 1904; Jones 1924). Subsequently, Mowrer described a successful behavioural intervention (bell and pad device) in nocturnal enuresis. Wolpe (1958) suggested, based on work in cats, that some states were antagonistic to anxiety (*ciprical inhibition*). He proposed that graded (imaginal) exposure to fear-evoking stimuli (*hierarchy* of fears), with simultaneous evocation of an antagonistic state (relaxation), would lead to gradual reduction in the anxiety response (*systematic desensitisation).* Wolpe's work was influential. At the Maudsley Hospital, London, Eysenck, Rachman, Marks, Gelder and colleagues subsequently developed exposure treatments for phobic disorders. It became apparent that exposure in vivo was superior to exposure in imagination and, furthermore, that relaxation was not necessary (Marks 1978). A further development was the recognition that self-exposure (exposure in the absence of the therapist) was also powerful (Bourque and Ladouceur 1980), paving the way for incorporation of self-exposure tasks for 'homework' between sessions. The development of rigorous controlled trials led to the acceptance of behaviour therapy as established clinical practice for the treatment of phobic and obsessive-compulsive disorders (Marks, Hodgson and Rachman 1975).

ELEMENTS OF BEHAVIOUR THERAPY

As described above, behaviour therapy in Britain evolved largely in the treatment of anxiety disorders. Evidence for its efficacy in the treatment of agoraphobia and obsessive-compulsive disorder (OCD) is well established (see below). This section therefore describes the elements of behaviour therapy for the treatment of anxiety disorders, although the general principles can be applied to most behaviours.

In BT, a key problem behaviour is identified and assessed and a specific treatment plan is agreed with the patient. Careful thorough assessment is essential because it not only helps decide if the presenting problem is suitable for BT, it also provides the outline for subsequent treatment.

The Assessment Interview

The assessment of the patient has three broad aims:

- definition of the core problem and associated factors

- engagement of the patient
- establishment of baseline measures.

Problem Definition

Assessment defines the behaviour, why it occurs (the patient's feared consequence if he or she does not act in this way), when it occurs and factors that modify it (see Figure 6.1). Avoidant and excessive behaviour are also noted. It is crucial to document avoidant behaviour as avoidances provide the basis for exposure. Avoidant behaviour is usually all pervasive, but often only becomes apparent on direct questioning. For example, a subject who is phobic about vomiting may readily volunteer that TV programmes with a medical theme are avoided for fear of seeing vomit. More subtle avoidances (ensuring that food is eaten within sell-by dates, avoidance of 'unsafe' foods, crowded pubs, public toilets) and excesses (cleaning of work-surfaces with bleach several times a day, washing of hands excessively to avoid 'germs') may only become apparent on direct questioning. Modifying factors must also be noted. Use of alcohol, particularly in social phobics, carrying of 'talisman', which may range from benzodiazepine tablets to lucky charms, are important modifiers to ask about directly. Maintaining factors: misguided reassurance (and hence reinforcement) from relatives, inadvertent, often unconscious 'gains' from the behaviour (for example, avoidance of particular responsibilities because of the disability) must also tactfully be elicited as these contribute not only to treatment but also to motivation to improve. Mental state examination is also crucial. Depression is common in OCD and in social phobia and will need to be treated before embarking on BT. Psychotic beliefs may mimic OCD in presentation and must be assessed. Current medication and previous treatment are also important. It is always wise to check what exactly patients mean if they say they have had previous 'BT'. If they have had BT then determination of why it failed is important.

What is the behaviour?

Why does it occur?

When does it occur?

Where does it occur?

What makes it **better** or **worse?**

Talisman?

Avoidances? Excesses?

Maintaining/Perpetuating factors?

Mental state?

Figure 6.1 Crucial questions in assessment

Engagement

Engagement of the patient is crucial in most forms of BT. Explanation of the behavioural model to the patients will allow them to understand the rationale for treatment, help them to develop their own targets in treatment, and, most importantly, by providing an explanation for the treatment, maximise their motivation to carry out behavioural tasks. Subjects are much more willing to carry out homework tasks and place themselves in anxiety-evoking situations if they can understand the rationale for doing so. Furthermore, often simply explaining the process of their fear, as described below, leads to reduction in anxiety as they begin to understand how components of their anxiety interact.

(a) *Explaining the symptoms.* Lang's three systems model of behaviour (Lang 1971) provides a useful outline for explanation (Figure 6.2). Lang's three-systems model describes three key components of behaviour: **A**ffect (feelings – here including physical and mental), **B**ehaviour and **C**ognitions. Use of

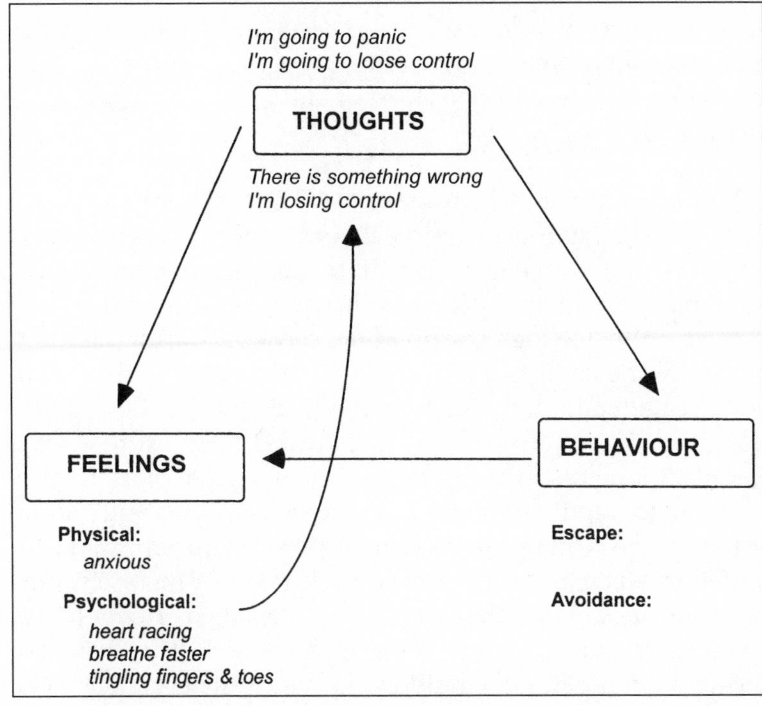

Figure 6.2 Lang's three-systems model of behaviour

the subject's *own symptoms* of anxiety and behaviour, in their own words, personalises the model and increases its relevance for them. The example shown applies to agoraphobia but can obviously be adapted to most disorders. In this example, subjects first think 'I'm going to panic and lose control'. They immediately feel anxious. Questioning revealed physical symptoms: heart racing, feeling short of breath and tingling in their hands and around their mouth. This in turn increased their anxiety and made them feel they would collapse and lose control. Recognition of this connection between thoughts and feelings is often a revelation to these subjects who, for the first time realise, how their symptoms may interact to compound their anxiety. As their anxiety increases, the subjects usually escape from the situation, generally with a rapid and dramatic reduction in anxiety. This behaviour reinforces their belief that they would have lost control and panicked. It also reinforces their anxiety when they next come in contact with the feared situation or object. Avoidant behaviour has a similar effect.

(b) *Outlining the treatment rationale.* The therapist explains that, in the behavioural approach, one concentrates primarily on the behavioural component of the model, interrupting the viscious circle at this point, with changes in thoughts, and subsequently feelings, responding secondarily to this. Emphasis on the cognitive arm will vary according to the condition treated and the exact methods employed (see under Cognitive Therapy: A New Departure?). Exposure to the feared situation is then discussed. The principle of *habituation* – the gradual reduction in fear if one stays in the feared situation, and the waning of the fear response with repeated presentation – is explained. Grading (rating on a hierarchy) the exposure tasks, and the necessity of repeated, frequent exposure *until the anxiety reduces* is discussed. The first step chosen by the patient should evoke some anxiety for it to be useful – a degree of anxiety the subject can just manage.

Throughout these explanations, use of diagrams shared with the subject, involvement of the subject in drawing the diagrams, writing down symptoms, all emphasise the importance of the patient's involvement in treatment and begins to transfer the focus of control and decision making to the patient – an important introduction to a behavioural approach.

(c) *Describing the structure of BT sessions.* BT is a focused structured treatment and it is important that the subject is aware of this. One explains that treatment will initially be weekly, possibly fortnightly. Subjects will be expected to generate and carry out homework tasks between sessions, with written diaries of their progress. Each session will last about 45 minutes with the agenda set at the beginning of each session – generally review of homework, discussion of particular issues, problems and setting of new targets. A number of treatment sessions (usually 10) is agreed with a plan to review progress at that point.

Establishment of Baseline Measurements

Precise measurement of patient's difficulties are important for three reasons:

1 They help assessment by defining the degree of difficulty.
2 They are useful during treatment to allow measurement of progress.
3 They serve as encouragement to patients in treatment – subjects often forget the enormity of their problem when they first presented.

There are numerous rating scales, inventories and checklists available. Measurement can be specific for the disorder, e.g. the Maudsley Obsessive-Compulsive Inventory or the Yale–Brown Obsessive-Compulsive Scale. General ratings of difficulty of goals and problems is also important. We use a 0–8 point scale to rate severity of presenting problem and targets – both therapist and subject rate this as there may be a divergence of opinion which may be used in treatment. Impact of the disorder on the subject's functioning is also rated. These ratings are then used throughout treatment to monitor progress and to provide feedback for the subject.

At the end of assessment, the therapist should know whether or not the problem is suitable for BT, and the client should understand the rationale and mechanism for BT. Baseline measures of symptoms severity and impact on functioning of the disorder should be established. The next step is to construct an outline for treatment.

The Treatment Schedule

The first step in outlining a treatment plan is to define the problem clearly. Establishment of clear goals is also important – it is not enough to say 'I don't want to be afraid in public' as this is both unrealistic and non-specific. Establishment of clear, realistic relevant goals focuses the subject on improvement, provides tangible end-points which can be readily measured, and will be relevant to the subject's every-day life, e.g. to go the supermarket on my own twice a week, to travel by tube to work every day, to go to the cinema with friends once a week. Once end of treatment goals have been established, one can then use them to construct mini-goals (targets) for each week. As described earlier, treatment involves exposure to the feared situation or object with prevention of the subject's usual responses. Exposure should be prolonged (to allow habituation to occur), focused, realistic and repeated often until the anxiety is reduced to an acceptable level. Exposure should not just be direct exposure to the object/situation, it should also include 'indirect exposure' by tackling avoidances built into the subject's everyday life. Prevention of the patient's usual response to exposure must often be dealt with by breaking the behaviour down into several components and tackling each piece in turn – e.g. in hand-washing to initially agree to reduce from washing to the shoulder, to the elbow, wrist, etc., and then to tackle the number of repeated hand washes and so on. Involvement of family members as 'co-therapists' is often helpful.

COGNITIVE THERAPY: A NEW DEPARTURE?

The above schedule outlines a behavioural approach to disorders. A cognitive approach to problems has been hailed as a 'new departure', with great discussion in the literature of the distinction between cognitive therapy (CT) and behaviour therapy (BT). In some cases, the debate is academic. Awareness of the importance of cognitions is an integral part of BT. While the focus of treatment is on behaviour, it is realised that cognitions influence behaviour, and equally that behaviour influences cognitions. Part of the effect of exposure is the negation of the patients' underlying beliefs that they will, for example, faint, collapse, or lose control in response to exposure to the feared situation. In BT, the emphasis is on changing behaviour with recognition that changes in cognitions and, subsequently, emotions will follow (although often with a considerable time lapse – so called 'cognitive lag'). There are, nonetheless, key differences between CT and BT, in particular in CT as originally described for depression (Beck et al 1979).

CT: Origins and Evolution

Despite behaviour therapy's success in treating phobic and obsessive-compulsive disorders, there remained a significant number of disorders in which behaviour therapy had little or no effect. A key disorder was depression; key by virtue of its importance in general psychiatry. Pure behavioural techniques had not proved effective in depression. A successful psychological approach to the disorder was still lacking and it was onto this fertile ground that the seeds of *Cognitive Behaviour Therapy* (CT) fell.

Beck postulated that systematic errors in thinking underlie at least some forms of depression (Beck et al 1979). These errors include selective attention to negative features of a situation, magnification of the catastrophic implications of these situations and arbitrary inferences, i.e. the drawing of conclusions (usually pessimistic) not based on the data available. These patterns of thinking give rise to the 'negative triad' – a negative view of the self, the future and the world. Underlying these negative automatic thoughts (NATs) are schemata – internal models used to organise perception and govern and evaluate behaviour. Some schemata are helpful; others are dysfunctional. Beck suggests that a critical incident may lead to activation of these dysfunctional schemata, particularly when the critical incident is congruent with the dysfunctional assumption. This prompts a surge of related NATs which are associated with negative emotions and which promote depressed mood. The core aim of treatment is to make the subject aware of the NATs, challenge them and replace them with more realistic and appropriate thoughts. More recently, recognition of the dysfunctional core beliefs and their origin and restructuring of these core 'schemata' has become a further aim in treatment. Many of the processes in treatment are behavioural – keeping of a (cognitive) diary, behavioural experiments to test out the validity of the beliefs, keeping a diary of activity, scheduling acts of mastery and pleasure, etc. As in BT, engagement of the patient and a focus on patient-led treatment, regular homework and structured sessions are important. Beck himself acknowledges the behavioural contribution to CT (Beck 1993). The core thrust of treatment, however, is on cognitions, with the belief that focus on changing cognitions will lead to improvement in depressed mood and alteration in behaviour.

CT: New Solutions, New Difficulties

The Beckian model for depression is clearly different from a behavioural approach. One could argue, however, that CT for other disorders (for example, social phobia and obsessive-compulsive disorder) are less clearly distinct from BT (Salkovskis and Kirk 1989), retaining large components of BT (although the two have diverged more with time (Salkovskis and Kirk 1997)). It is also important to realise, both when people offer to provide CT for patients and when reading about clinical trials of CT, that the term CT has become much less well defined. Beck has developed his model to include treatment of anxiety disorders and, more recently, personality disorders (Beck 1991). Widely differing treatment approaches such as 'schema-focused therapy' (Padesky 1994) or a package incorporating social skills training and problem-solving skills can be included under the rubric 'CT'. This imprecision in what constitutes CT leads to difficulties in analysing effects and components of CT. There are other, theoretical, difficulties with the model.

Beck's model and treatment approach are based on detailed careful clinical observation. It stresses the links between cognition and emotion – a concept in agreement with cognitive psychology. It is not, however, based on scientific observation and has developed independently of, and distinct from, cognitive psychology – a distinction that troubles many (Teasdale 1993). Some of the difficulties in CT are well summarised by Teasdale: similar changes in cognitions arise when depression is successfully treated with antidepressants, recovered depressives do not show any evidence of persistent dysfunctional schemata, and there is a consistent lack of correlation between shift in cognitive beliefs and response to treatment. Furthermore, rational argument is frequently ineffective in changing emotions. A further development has been the recent finding in a large sample of depressed individuals that 'full CT', as described by Beck, was no more effective either at the end of treatment or at six month follow-up than the behavioural activation component of CT or schema-focused therapy (Jacobson et al 1996). Interestingly, while CT for depression is faced with increasing questions, the development of the principles of CT for other disorders has been very successful. One such example is the CT model for panic (Clark 1986).

Conclusion

Cognitive therapy has provided a new impetus for research and development in the psychological therapies. The focus on the interplay between cognitions and emotions makes intuitive sense and is supported by cognitive psychology. Initial clinical studies of cognitive therapy, while problematic, are promising (see below).

EFFICACY OF INTERVENTION

Phobias

Behavioural intervention is generally effective in *specific phobia* – clinically significant improvement is achieved in 70–85% of cases (Emmelkamp 1982; Marks 1987 – for review see Emmeklamp 1994). In common with other anxiety disorders, in vivo exposure, with prolongation of exposure until anxiety begins to reduce significantly, appears to be the most effective component of treatment (Marshall 1988). In *blood-injury phobia* applied tension techniques combined with exposure gives better results than simple exposure (Ost, Sterner and Fellenius 1989). A number of studies have demonstrated significant effects of in vivo exposure for *social phobia* (Butler et al 1984; Mattick and Peters 1988; Turner, Beidel and Jacob 1994). While there is evidence that cognitive behavioural interventions, combined with exposure therapy, can be effective (Butler et al 1984; Mattick and Peters 1988), and that combining cognitive interventions with exposure may be more effective than exposure alone, this remains controversial (Hope, Heimberg and Bruch 1990; Scholing and Emmelkamp 1993; Hope, Heimberg and Bruch 1995). Marked reduction of *agoraphobic* symptoms by live exposure has been documented in dozens of controlled studies – for review see Mattick et al (1990). These effects appears to be maintained: in 10 studies reviewed by O'Sullivan and Marks (1990) – with a mean follow-up period four years – 76% of patients were improved or much improved with 24% rated as unimproved. However, it must be pointed out that while significant improvements are achieved, many patients experience residual symptoms (Jacobson 1988). Combining cognitive treatment with exposure for agoraphobia appears no more effective than exposure alone (Chambless and Gillis 1993). Cognitive treatment for panic is based on a model of catastrophic misinterpretation of physical symptoms. Cognitive therapy has been found to be more effective than imipramine (Clark et al 1994) and applied relaxation (Clark et al 1994; Beck et al 1994; Ost and Westling 1995). The specificity of the treatment has been questioned by Shear et al (1994) who found no significant differences between CT and a control therapy (reflective listening) in 45 patients with panic. Most of these trials focused on patients with panic alone, or with mild–moderate degrees of agoraphobia. Patients with severe agoraphobia respond less well to cognitive intervention alone, with good response to exposure prompting some authors to suggest that exposure remains the treatment of choice for this group (Beck et al 1994).

Summary

The efficacy of behavioural intervention in phobic states has been clearly demonstrated. There is some evidence to suggest that cognitive techniques may improve outcome in social phobia and panic disorders. However, exposure treatment appears essential in panic disorder with severe agoraphobia.

Obsessive-Compulsive Disorder

Compulsive ritualisers respond well to live exposure and response prevention (Marks 1987). Between 70 and 80% of patients who accept and comply with treatment will improve (Perse 1988). Gains tend to persist over several years (Ost 1989). In general, modelling of exposure does not enhance outcome (Rachman, Hodgson and Marks 1973). While exposure to obsessional ruminations (for example, through use of a loop-tape) is also feasible, behavioural intervention is less successful in these patients (Marks 1987). Foa (1979) has suggested that treatment failure in OCD is linked to patients attitudes and beliefs about their symptoms. Cognitive therapists have developed cognitive models for OCD (Salkovskis 1989). Emmelkamp and colleagues contrasted the efficacy of behavioural (exposure) and cognitive-behavioural (exposure with self-instruction; rational emotive therapy; and rational emotive therapy with exposure) interventions in OCD (Emmelkamp et al 1980; Emmelkamp, Visser and Hoekstra 1988). Treatments gave equivalent outcomes. It should be noted, however, that many of the 'cognitive' interventions included exposure. Van Oppen compared exposure and cognitive therapy (Foa, Davidson and Rothbaum 1995), and both treatments led to significant improvements. Again, however, the cognitive component entailed exposure (behavioural experiments to test the validity of their beliefs).

Summary

Exposure and response prevention, standard behavioural interventions, remain the gold standard for OCD, with well-maintained treatment response in 70–80% of patients. Early work on cognitive interventions is promising, but as yet trials remain scant. Furthermore, while most cognitive treatments in OCD focus on content and meaning of beliefs, most cognitive interventions incorporate exposure.

Depression

A number of investigators have documented the usefulness of cognitive therapy in depression . Key studies in the assessment of CT in depression include the NIMH study (Elkin et al 1985), the University of Minnesota study of CT and pharmacotherapy (Evans et al 1992), the University of Pittsburgh Study (Kupfer et al 1992; Frank et al 1991), and the second Sheffield Psychotherapy Project (Shapiro et al 1994). Key difficulties exist in the design and methodology of many of the studies outlined by Hollon, Shelton and Loosen (1991). *What Works for Whom? A Critical Review of Psychotherapy Research* provides detailed summaries of the major trials in CT (Roth and Fenagy 1996). The editors draw a number of conclusions from the multitude of research carried out to date in CT in depression:

1 CT appears to be effective in acute depression.
2 Evidence for the superiority of combination treatments over psychological intervention alone is weak.
3 Evidence does not suggest that CT is more effective than medical treatment.
4 While there is some evidence to suggest that CT may reduce the risk of relapse in depression, the absence of long-term follow-up in most trials makes this difficult to assess with confidence.

Other Conditions

Difficulties in engaging and motivating patients with **anorexia nervosa** frequently limit the use of behavioural techniques in this condition. Behavioural interventions have, however, been used. Crisp et al (1991) used behavioural techniques in an in-patient treatment package compared with out-patient psychodynamic or group therapy. While in-patient treatment initially resulted in greater gains, subsequent greater relapse rates in this group led to the supremacy of the out-patient interventions. Treasure et al (1995) contrasted cognitive analytic therapy with educational-behavioural treatment. There were no significant differences between the two groups on measures of weight gain although the CAT group reported greater subjective improvement. There is little reliable evidence for the efficacy of exposure and response prevention alone in *bulimia nervosa*. Although there are relatively few controlled trials of CT for bulimia nervosa, results are encouraging. Wilson and Fairburn (1993) report a mean percentage reduction in binge eating of 73–93%, and in purging of 77–94%; however, mean remission rates were lower – 51–71% for binge eating and 36–56% for purging. A review by Craighead and Agras (1991) provides similar findings. Exposure in *post-traumatic stress disorder* has met with mixed success – improvement in PTSD symptoms but little change in depression and anxiety (Foa, Davidson and Rothbaum 1995). Studies by Foa and colleagues comparing exposure, 'stress inoculation training' and a combination of both suggest that all treatments are equally effective (Foa, Davidson and Rothbaum 1995; Foa et al 1991). Behavioural techniques such as operant conditioning, social skills training, distraction, exposure have met with limited success in the treatment of psychotic symptoms in *schizophrenia* (for review, see Sellwood et al (1994). Development of cognitive-behavioural interventions (identifying stressors, enhancing patients skills in controlling cues and their reactions to them) has met with some success (Tarrier et al 1993). Drury et al (in press) report improvement in subjects with non-affective psychosis treated with a cognitive-behavioural package comprising individual and group cognitive therapy, family psycho-education and support and behavioural activation. The usefulness of these techniques is limited by high refusals to enter treatments, and high drop-out rates. The paucity of clinical trials means that cognitive-behavioural techniques in schizophrenia, while promising, have yet to be adequately tested.

CONCLUSIONS

Behaviour therapy (BT) is an effective treatment for anxiety disorders, in particular phobias and obsessive-compulsive disorder. A significant (70–80%) proportion of patients can be expected to improve, with maintenance of gains. Cognitive therapy (CT) has provided new developments and ideas, particularly in the treatment of depression. In many cases, cognitive therapy includes a significant behavioural approach. The term 'Cognitive therapy' has evolved to included a variety of approaches, and a definition of what is meant by cognitive therapy should be sought before embarking on treatment and when interpreting clinical trials. Current research suggests that new assessment of the interplay between cognitions and emotions, and behavioural and cognitive components of treatment, will provide impetus for further developments and successes in the psychological treatment of psychiatric disorders.

REFERENCES

Ayllon T & Azrin N (1968) *The Token Economy* Wiley: New York

Beck AT, Rush AJ, Shaw BF & Emery G (1979) *Cognitive Therapy of Depression: A Treatment Manual* Guilford Press: New York

Beck AT (1991) Cognitive therapy: a 30-year retrospective *Am Psycholog* **46**(4): 368–75

Beck AT (1993) *Cognitive Therapy of Depression: A Personal Reflection* Scottish Cultural Press: Aberdeem

Beck JG, Stanley MA, Baldwin LE, Deagle EA & Averill PM (1994) Comparison of cognitive therapy and relaxation training for panic disorder *J Consult Clin Psychol* **62**: 818–26

Bourque P & Ladouceur R (1980) An investigation of various performance-based treatments with acrophobics *Behav Res Ther* **18**: 161–70

Butler G, Cullington A, Mumby M, Amies P & Gelder M (1984) Exposure and anxiety management in the treatment of social phobia *J Consult Clinl Psychol* **52**: 642–50

Chambless DL & Gillis MM (1993) Cognitive therapy of anxiety disorders *J Consult Clin Psychol* **61**: 248–60

Clark DM (1986) A cognitive approach to panic *Behav Res Ther* **24**: 461–70

Clark DM, Salkovskis PM, Hackmann A, Middleton H, Anastasiades P & Gelder M (1994) A comparison of cognitive therapy, applied relaxation and imipramine in the treatment of panic disorder *Br J Psychiat* **164**: 759–69

Craighead LW & Agras W (1991) Mechansims of action in cognitive-behavioural and pharmocological interventions for obesity and bulimia nervosa *J Consult Clin Psychol* **59**: 115–25

Crisp AH, Norton K, Gowers S, Halek C, Bowyer C, Yeldham D, Levett G & Bhat A (1991) A controlled study of the effect of therapies aimed at adolescent and family psychopathology in anorexia nervosa *Br J Psychiat* **159**: 325–33

Davey GCL (1992) Classical conditioning and the acquistion of human fears and phobias: a review and synthesis of the literature *Adv Behav Res Ther* **14**: 29–66

Drury V, Birchwood M, Cochrane R & Macmillan F (in press) Cognitive therapy and recovery from acute psychosis: a controlled trial I: Impact on psychotic symptoms *Br J Psychiat* (In Press)

Elkin I, Parloff MB, Hadley SW & Autry JH (1985) NIMH treatment of depression collaborative research program *Arch Gen Psychiat* **42**: 305–16

Emmelkamp PMG, van der Helm M, van Zanten BL & Plochg I (1980) Treatment of obsessive-compulsive patients: The contribution of self-instructional training to the effectiveness of exposure *Behav Res Ther* **18**: 61–6

Emmelkamp PMG (1982) *Phobic and Obsessive Compulsive Disorders: Theory, Research and Practice* Plenum Press: New York

Emmelkamp PMG, Visser S & Hoekstra RJ (1988) Cognitive therapy vs exposure in-vivo in the treatment of obsessive-compulsive disorder *Cognitive Ther Res* **12**: 103–14

Emmelkamp PMG (1994) Behaviour therapy with adults. In AE Bergin & SL Garfield (eds) *Handbook of Psychotherapy and Behaviour Change* Wiley: New York

Evans MD, Hollon SD, DeRubeis RJ, Piasecki JM, Grove WM, Garvey MJ & Tuason VB (1992) Differential relapse following cognitive therapy and pharmacotherapy for depression *Arch Gen Psychiat* **49**: 802–8

Foa EB (1979) Failure on treating obsessive-compulsives. *Behav Res Ther* **17**: 169–76

Foa EB, Rothbaum BO, Riggs DS & Murdoch TB (1991) Treatment of PTSD in rape victims: a comparison between cognitive-behavioural procedures and counselling *J Consult Clin Psychol* **59**: 715–23

Foa EB, Davidson J & Rothbaum BO (1995) Treatment of post-traumatic stress disorder. In GO Gabbard (ed) *Treatment of Psychiatric Disorders : The DSM-IV Edition* American Psychiatric Press: Washington, DC

Frank E, Prien RF, Jarrett RB, Keller MB, Kupfer DJ, Lavori PW, Rush J & Weissman MM (1991) Conceptualization and rationale for consensus definitions of terms in major depressive disorder *Arch Gen Psychiat* **48**: 851–5

Hollon SD, Shelton RC & Loosen PT (1991) Cognitive therapy and pharmacotherapy for depression *J Consult Clin Psychol* **59**(1): 88–99

Hope DA, Heimberg RG & Bruch MA (1990) *The Importance of Cognitive Interventions in the Treatment of Social Phobia* Phobia Society of America: Washington, DC

Hope DA, Heimberg RG & Bruch MA (1995) Dismantling cognitive-behavioural group therapy for social phobia *Behav Res Ther* **33**: 637–50

Jacobson NS, Wilson L & Tupper C (1988) The clinical significance of treatment gains resulting from exposure-based interventions for agoraphobia: a re-analysis of outcome data *Behav Ther* **10**: 133–45

Jacobson NS, Dobson KS, Truax PA, Koerner K, Gollan JK, Gortner E & Prince SE (1996) A component analysis of cognitive behavioural treatment for depression *J Consult Clin Psychol* **64**: 295–304

Jones MC (1924) Elimination of children's fears *J Expt Psychol* **7**: 382–97

Kupfer DJ, Frank E, Perel JM, Corens C, Mallinger AG, Thase ME

Lang PG (1971) The application of psychophysiological methods to the study of psychotherapy and behaviour modification. In Bergin & Garfield (eds) *Handbook of Psychotherapy and Behavioural Change* Wiley: New York pp 75–125

Marks IM, Hodgson R & Rachman S (1975) Treatment of chronic obsessive-compulsive neurosis by in-vivo exposure *Br J Psychiat* **127**: 349–64

Marks IM (1978) Exposure treatments. In S Agras (ed) *Behaviour Modification* (2nd edition) Little Brown: Boston pp 163–242

Marks IM (1987) *Fears, Phobias and Rituals* Oxford University Press: Oxford

Marshall WL (1988) Behavioural indices of habituation and sensitisation during exposure to phobic stimuli *Behav Res Ther* **26**: 67–77

Mattick RP & Peters L (1988) Treatment of severe social phobia: effects of guided exposure with and without cognitive restructuring *J Consult Clin Psychol* **56**: 251–60

Mattick RP, Andrews G, Hadzi-Pavlovic D & Christensen H (1990) Treatment of pani and agoraphobia: an integrative review *J Nerv Ment Dis* **178**: 567–76

Mowrer OH (1960) *Learning Theory and Behaviour* Wiley: New York

O'Sullivan G & Marks IM (1990) Long-term outcome of phobic and obsessive-compulsive disorders after treatment. In R Noyes, M Roth & GD Burrows (eds) *The Treatment of Anxiety*Elsevier: Amsterdam

Ost LG (1989) A maintenance programme for behavioural treatment of anxiety disorders *Behav Res Ther* **27**: 123–30

Ost LG, Sterner U & Fellenius J (1989) Applied tension, applied relaxation in the treatment of blood phobia *Behav Res Ther* **27**: 109

Ost LG & Westling BE (1995) Applied relaxation vs cognitive behaviour therapy in the treatment of panic disorder *Behav Res Ther* **55**: 145–58

Padesky CA (1994) Schema change process in cognitive therapy *Clin Psychol Psychother* **1**(5): 267–78

Perse T (1988) Obsessive-compulsive disorder: a treatment review . *J Clin Psychiat* **49**: 48–55

Rachman S, Hodgson R & Marks IM (1973) Treatment of OCD by modelling and flooding in vivo *Behav Res Ther* **11**: 463–71

Rachman S (1991) Neo-conditioning and the classical theory of fear acquisition *Clin Psychol Rev* **11**: 155–73

Roth A & Fenagy P (1996) *What Works for Whom? A Critical Review of Psychotherapy Research* Guildford Press: New York

Salkovskis PM (1989) Obsessions and compulsions. In J Scott, JMG Williams & AT Beck (eds) *Cognitive Therapy: A Clinical Casebook* Croom Helm: London

Salkovskis PM & Kirk J (1989) Obsessional disorders. In K Hawton, PM Salkovskis, J Kirk & DM Clark (eds) *Cognitive Behaviour*

Therapy for Psychiatric Problems: A Practical Guide Oxford University Press: Oxford pp 129–69

Salkovskis PM & Kirk J (1997) Obsessive-compulsive disorder. In DM Clark & CG Fairburn (eds) *Science and Practice of Cognitive Behaviour Therapy* Oxford Medical Publications: Oxford pp 179–209

Scholing A & Emmelkamp PMG (1993) Exposure with and without cognitive therapy for generalized social phobia: effects of individual and group treatment *Behav Res Ther* **31**: 667–81

Sellwood W, Haddock G, Tarrier N & Yusupoff L (1994) Advances in the psychological management of positive symptoms of schizophrenia *Internat Rev Psychiat* **6**: 201–15

Shapiro DA, Barkham M, Rees A, Hardy GE, Reynolds S & Startup M (1994) Effects of treatment duration and severity of depression on the effectiveness of cognitive-behavioural and psychodynamic-interpersonal psychotherapy *J Consult Clin Psychol* **62**(3): 522–34

Shear MK, Pilkonis PA, Cloitrem M & Leon AC (1994) Cognitive behavioural treatment compared with non-prescriptive treatment of panic disorder *Arch Gen Psychiat* **51**: 395–401

Tarrier N, Beckett R, Harwood S, Baker A, Yusupoff L & Ugarterburu I (1993) A trial of two cognitive-behavioural methods of treating drug-resistant residual psychotic symptoms in schizophrenic patients I: Outcome *Br J Psychiat* **162**: 524–32

Teasdale JD (1993) Emotion and two kinds of meaning *Behav Res Ther* **31**: 339–54

Treasure J, Todd G, Brolly M, Tiller J, Nehmed A & Denman F (1995) A pilot study of a randomised trial of cognitive analytical therapy versus educational behavioural therapy for adult anorexia nervosa. *Behav Res Ther* **33**: 363–7

Turner SM, Beidel DC & Jacob RG (1994) Social phobia: a comparison of behaviour therapy and atenolol *J Consult Clin Psychol* **62**: 350–8

Wilson GT & Fairburn CG (1993) Cognitive treatments for eating disorders *J Consult Clin Psychol* **61**: 261–9

Wolpe J (1958) *Psychotherapy by Reciprocal Inhibition* Stanford University Press: Stanford

CHAPTER 7

Electroconvulsive Therapy

Gerald O'Mahony

St Bartholomew's Hospital, London

and

Michael J. Travis

Institute of Psychiatry, London

INTRODUCTION

Electroconvulsive therapy (ECT) is an effective treatment for a range of mental illnesses. Its main use is in the acute treatment of major depressive illness, whether a single or recurrent episode. It is an effective treatment for mood disturbance in bipolar affective disorder, major depression, mania or mixed affective state, and it has a particular role in the treatment of depression in pregnancy and puerperal psychosis (Miller 1994). ECT may be indicated in the prophylactic treatment of major depressive illness. It may have a role in the treatment of schizophrenia in which it has a specific indication in the treatment of catatonic states. It is suggested to be of benefit in Parkinson's disease and in neuroleptic malignant syndrome, though it does not have a role in the routine management of either of these. The efficacy of ECT in the treatment of mood disorders is supported by an extensive literature and

Understanding Psychiatric Treatment. Edited by G. O'Mahony and J.V. Lucey.

experience of those who use it. Nonetheless, its application after close to 60 years remains contentious.

BACKGROUND

The introduction of ECT in the 1930s came at a time when development of treatment strategies was not constrained by regulatory bodies, peer review or an informed public. A body of knowledge accumulated which allowed for modification of its indications and its practical administration. ECT was a logical development of convulsive therapy first credited in the modern era to Meduna in 1934. The use of therapeutic induction of seizures was based upon theoretical grounds and an earlier literature. Clinical observation of patients with coincidental epilepsy suggested that improvements in mental state occurred at times of seizure activity. The rapid progression from hypothesis to ECT's introduction as a treatment method was congruent with an atmosphere of therapeutic optimism in relation to the development of physical treatments: Wagner-Jauregg's malarial fever therapy for syphilitic general paralysis of the insane (1917), Sakels insulin coma therapy (1933) and Moniz' psycho-surgery (1935) (Abrams 1994). This temporal placement fashioned subsequent events by allowing the development of the treatment to a point improbable in the ethics of the modern era. ECT was associated firmly in the public and professional mind with contemporaneous therapeutic strategies. Malaria treatment was superseded, insulin coma abandoned and psycho-surgery re-evaluated, restricted and refined to a rarity. Understandably ECT has not escaped scepticism. Progress towards de-institutionalisation has been accompanied by a broadening of the debate on treatment. Refusal to accept previous orthodoxy has encouraged questioning of the validity or appropriateness of physical treatments in isolation. Since recognition of psychological, social antecedents and perpetuating factors of mental disorder is essential in treatment planning, the adoption of ECT as a treatment strategy appears counter-intuitive. Early expectation was for ECT to be effective in the treatment of schizophrenia. Later experience showed its prime use to be in the treatment of affective disorders.

CLINICAL INDICATIONS AND EFFICACY

Depressive Disorders

This is the most common indication for ECT. A series of reviews detail its effectiveness in depressive disorders (Kendell 1981; Fink 1979). The advent of antidepressant medications, the tricyclic antidepressants (TCA) and mono amine oxidase inhibitors (MOAI) from the mid 1950s led to a reappraisal of the place of ECT in the treatment of depression. Response rates to ECT (71%) compared favourably to imipramine 100–200 mg daily for four weeks (52%) and phenelzine 30–60 mg daily for four weeks (30%) and placebo (39%) in studies conducted by the Medical Research Council (Weschler, Grosser and Greenblatt 1965). Furthermore, half the patients not responding to tricyclic antidepressants recovered after a subsequent course of ECT (MRC Clinical Psychiatry Committee 1965). However, the consistent findings of research showing an initial response rate of 70% to ECT has not won unquestioned acceptance (Nobler and Sackheim 1994).

The confounding variables of study design, case acquisition, selection criteria, lack of operationally defined treatment groups, inadequacies of controls and problems in ensuring subject and rater blindness to the procedure; have made meta-analysis of studies problematic. The equation has been complicated by the introduction of lithium augmentation, consideration of the place of mood stabilisers in the treatment of affective disorders and the more recent introduction of the SSRIs. The development of effective pharmacotherapy for depressive illness has progressively reduced the application of ECT, now more likely employed in depressive illness resistant to antidepressant medication and in patient groups in whom ECT may be the treatment of choice, such as the elderly

(Nobler and Sackheim 1994; Benbow 1995). The use of ECT in England dropped by about one-third in the nine years to 1989 (Pippard 1992). The available data points to high response rates of 60% or more to oral antidepressants when given in appropriate doses for sufficient time (Dinan 1998), choice of antidepressants being determined by tolerability, safety, side-effect profile and cost. ECT is now more likely to be employed in treatment resistance or in patients who require rapid onset of symptomatic relief. It is indicated for those with life-threatening illness, those with active suicidal intent, those unable to tolerate oral treatment, or for whom ECT has previously proven of benefit. In the Northwick Park ECT Trial (Clinical Research Centre 1984) prospectively randomised depressed patients received either real ECT or mock ECT, antidepressants were withheld during the initial course of ECT/simulated ECT, patients and raters were blind to the group they entered. Patients received modified ECT (anaesthesia and ECT) or sham ECT with induction of anaesthesia but no ECT stimulus. The trial showed that the most significant and only consistant predictor of response to ECT in depressed patients was the presence of delusions. This trial and a later study adopting a similar methodology (The Leicester trial, Brandon et al 1984) both showed significant benefits with real ECT. A combined analysis of the Northwick Park and Leicester trials (Buchan et al 1992) established that the response to ECT was real and not an elaborate placebo response. Patients were assessed by standardised interview schedules employing the Present State Examination (PSE) and Hamilton Depression Rating Scale (HDRS). Both studies concluded that ECT gave substantial benefit to deluded patients. The presence of retardation, particularly subjective anergia, slowness and under-activity and slowness of speech was predictive of response in the Leicester trial. Real ECT did not seem to benefit non-retarded and non-deluded patients. ECT benefited both those with delusions and retardation. Retardation appeared the most significant variable, the presence of delusions with retardation led to a greater response than retardation alone. While benefits are apparent at one month, this is not maintained by six months. A single successful course of ECT does not decrease the likelihood of future episodes of depression. At least half of the patients treated with ECT alone will relapse within two weeks of cession of ECT (Barton, Mehta and Snaith 1973). Current practice is therefore to prescribe an antidepressant concurrently with the course of ECT and maintain the patient on anti-depressants for at least six months after recovery. Relapse rates may be as high as 73% in some patient groups despite adequate medication (Godber et al 1987; Sackheim 1994).

Clinical Practice

The decision to prescribe ECT is influenced by the presenting level of distress and previous history of response to treatment. The typical progression is through a trial of oral antidepressants with introduction of ECT if response to treatment is not obtained. Definitions of adequate trials of treatment vary. Protocols using TCAs suggest that therapeutic dose levels should be maintained for at least six weeks with further incremental increase in non-responders to maximum tolerated dosage. Consideration of augmentation therapies comes next, or change to another class of drug such as an SSRI, or combining classes of drugs (Bridges, Hodgkiss and Malizia 1995). With the variety of suggested options across and between classes of drugs, a time course extending over many weeks is theoretically possible. In practice, this is not done. Depression is distressing for patients, relatives and health professionals involved in care. Prolonged hospitalisation jeopardises relationships and employment. Delay in effective treatment may be regarded as an iatrogenic cause of morbidity (Bonner and Howard 1995). ECT may be neglected in those in whom it has been previously effective and this could contribute to suicide risk (Barraclough et al 1974). The American Psychiatric Association's task force on ECT accepts the presence of situations when ECT may be used prior to trials of psychotropic agents. Primary indications for ECT therapy are suggested (American Psychiatric Association 1990) as:

- where there is requirement for rapid response on either medical or psychiatric grounds
- when the risk of other treatments outweighs the risks of ECT
- when there is a history of poor drug response and/or history of good response to ECT in previous episodes
- when treatment is indicated by patient preference.

According to the special committee of the UK Royal College of Psychiatrists (1995), the best predicators of response to ECT are:

- the number of typical features of depressive illness
- depressive illness with psychotic features
- those who have failed to respond to antidepressants may recover with subsequent ECT.

Depressed patients for whom ECT is indicated include those most severely ill and distressed. Those with suicidal intent, those refusing or unable to eat or take fluids. ECT probably has a more rapid onset of action than antidepressant medication. Improvements are seen after one to four treatments (i.e. 1–10 days) compared with a minimum time of 10–14 days for antidepressants (Scott and Whalley 1993).

Prophylactic Treatment

The need for continuation of treatment with effective antidepressant therapy is well established in affective disorder. ECT is an exception among physical treatments in that it is commonly withdrawn once it achieves symptomatic benefit. Its prime role is in the acute management of illness. Prevention of relapse or recurrences is normally achieved by pharmacotherapy or pharmacotherapy in combination with psychotherapy. For some, through intolerance of medication, difficulty in maintaining compliance, good response to ECT in the acute episode, or through patient preference, prophylactic treatment with ECT may be indicated. Illness relapse may be defined as exacerbation of a continuing episode after initial symptomatic improvement. Treatment aimed at relapse prevention is termed *continuation* treatment. Illness recurrence is a new episode of illness following recovery that has lasted several months. Treatment aimed at preventing recurrence is termed *maintenance* treatment.

Continuation ECT for prophylaxis may be scheduled at one- to four-week intervals, depending upon patient response. There is little research evidence to guide practice. One case report of successful maintenance ECT extending over six years involved 400 ECT treatments (Barnes et al 1997).

The prospective trials at Northwick Park and Leicester showed treatment benefit from ECT was no longer detectable at six months follow-up. This is often quoted as a justification for not employing ECT. The current management of depression with oral medication dictates six months of treatment in full dose after recovery from first episode. Opinions vary on second or subsequent episodes. Prescribing trends are towards prolonged treatment periods to prevent relapse or recurrence. When treating elderly patients with recurring depression, common practice is to continue antidepressants indefinitely; employing a tolerated antidepressant or mood stabiliser or both in combination. An investigation of prophylaxis in a three-year follow-up outcome study of depressive episodes (Frank et al 1990), showed a clear response to continuing treatment in therapeutic doses with imipramine.

Mania

ECT appears to have a mood stabilising action. This is particularly evident in states of hypomanic and manic excitement. It is the treatment of choice in aroused patients at risk of exhaustion and dehydration. It is more rapidly active and safer than high dose neuroleptics; it may be used as an adjunct to medication, in slow or inadequate response. It is safe and well tolerated in these conditions. A review of 50 years' experience of the use of ECT in mania showed evidence of effectiveness in 80% of patients. This was felt to be a primary effect of treatment and not an effect of an induced organic confusional state (Mukherjee, Sackheim and Schnur 1994).

Schizophrenia

ECT was initially proposed as a treatment for schizophrenia. Cerletti first administered ECT in April 1938 to a 39-year-old man diagnosed as suffering from schizophrenia. The consensus from research is that ECT shows efficacy in acute schizophrenia but not in chronic schizophrenia or where negative symptoms are prominent. ECT may have a specific benefit for the catatonic type of schizophrenia.

Review of adjunctive treatments in schizophrenia, comparing pharmacotherapy and ECT, is problematic since studies are small with diverse designs. There is little significant evidence to suggest an effective adjunctive action; ECT appeared most therapeutic in affective symptoms related to schizophrenia (Johns and Thomson 1995). Traditionally, ECT is regarded as the treatment of choice for catatonic schizophrenia In a report of 28 cases of catatonia associated with both affective and schizophrenic disorders, those treated with ECT had greater than 80% resolution of symptoms regardless of diagnostic sub-groups (Rohland, Carroll and Jacoby 1993).

Other Psychiatric Disorders

ECT is effective in some cases of neuroleptic malignant syndrome (NMS); a rare but potentially fatal idiosyncratic reaction to antipsychotic medication (Davis et al 1991). Parkinson's disease is frequently associated with depression. When depressive symptoms are treated with ECT, it is commonly reported that motor symptoms improve.

Mechanism of Action

The induction of a generalised seizure may be necessary for the effects of ECT. A variety of physiological changes occur, including changes in regional brain blood flow and metabolism. There are neuro-endocrine and neuro-transmitter modulatory effects. Neuro-chemical research indicates that ECT has some effect on virtually every neuro-transmitter system, these include those mediated by antidepressant medication, the noradrenaline and serotonin (5HT) systems. ECT also has effects on the gamma amino butyric acid (GABA) system (which can be modulated by the anxiolytics, the benzodiazepines), and the dopamine system which is the primary neuro-transmitter influenced by conventional antipsychotic drugs.

The apparent effect of ECT on all these systems is to enhance neuro-transmission, which is compatible with theories of the mode of action of antidepressant medication. Conversely, ECT reduces transmission through the cholinergic system. Deficits in acetyl choline neuro-transmission have been implicated in the pathophysiology of dementia. It has been speculated that the short-term memory deficits associated with ECT may be secondary to its effects upon cholinergic mechanisms (Mann and Kapur 1994). ECT may exert its primary effect via second messenger systems. These are chemical pathways responsible for the mediation of many stimuli received by individual nerve cells. Second messenger systems are implicated in the mechanism of action of psychotropic medication such as lithium, which is used in the treatment of mood disorders. ECT itself has an anticonvulsant activity. It appears to share mood stabilising properties concordant with the therapeutic application of anticonvulsant medications such as carbamazapine and sodium valproate for affective disorders.

PRACTICAL ASPECTS

ECT use has been documented to be effective in the treatment of adolescents with mood disorder. It is rarely used in the UK for this group. There is no evidence that ECT is less effective or is associated with more adverse effects in those under the age of 18. It is well tolerated by the elderly. Frequently due to co-morbid physical illness and urgent need for treatment response, it is the treatment of choice. The young demonstrate a lower seizure threshold than the old; as do women compared to men. Those on treatment with psychotropic medication may have altered seizure threshold. Neuroleptics are associated with reduction of seizure threshold, which may be employed therapeutically by administering a single dose of oral neuroleptic 12 hours before therapy. Recently vigorous seizures in patients treated with SSRI have been reported. Incremental increases in the dose of electrical stimulus via stimulus dosing may be necessary. ECT does not expose patients to risk of developing epilepsy. By its anticonvulsant activity it may be necessary to increase stimulation over the length of a course of treatment to continue to induce a seizure. Treatment schedules normally allow for administration two or three times weekly, without major differences in response. ECT was at one time employed up to twice daily in the management of acute mania, although this is not current practice. Treatment courses vary from a single treatment to 12 or more. Longer courses may be required in the elderly.

Anaesthesia

Technically ECT is largely an anaesthetic procedure. All contra-indications are relative. Each case is assessed on an individual basis. There is a need to ensure fitness for general anaesthetic. Normal pre-operative procedures include physical examination, ECG and chest x-ray, full blood count and urea and electrolyte estimation. Protocols are established setting out standards of staff proficiency and suitably equipped facilities. ECG monitoring is standard. Resuscitation equipment must be available. Patients are fasted. The airway must be protected, especially for those at risk of aspiration. For the pregnant woman, prophylactic antacids are administered and intubation may be required. The patient is pre-oxygenated. This is because optimal oxygenation facilitates seizures and prepares the patient for the apnoeic phase of anaesthesia secondary to muscle relaxants. Those at high risk include patients with a recent myocardial infarction (MI); highest risk, 10 days post-MI. Three months post-MI, patients are at low risk. Raised intracranial pressure is a contraindication.

Physiological Aspects

There is marked autonomic nervous system stimulation with ECT. Initial parasympathetic drive leads to bradycardia (slowing of heart rate) and hypotension followed by sympathetic discharge with tachycardia and a pressor effect with transient increase of intracranial pressure. The presence of a cerebral space occupying lesion is a contraindication to ECT.

Electrode Placement

Bilateral electrode placement is currently favoured. Unilateral ECT application to the non-dominant cerebral hemisphere may be associated with less memory impairment, but may have a slower onset of action (Abrams et al 1983).

Side-Effects – Safety

The most commonly reported side-effect with ECT is memory loss; affecting virtually all patients. Short-term memory loss post-ECT is common. Assessment is complicated since memory deficits are common in depressive illness. Memory impairment is less frequent since the introduction of pulse wave ECT, superseding high energy sine wave ECT (Weiner et al 1986). Short-term anterograde amnesia is commonly associated with a post-ECT/anaesthesia confusional state. Side-effects are temporary. Three months after cessation of ECT there is no apparent impairment (Johnstone et al 1980). Calev et al (1991) reporting on the early and long-term effects of ECT and depression on memory and other cognitive functions, report significant impairment of memory function at the end of ECT therapy. By one month, performance returned to pre-treatment levels and exceeded pre-treatment levels by six months. Therefore, the therapeutic response to treatment of a depressive episode may be associated with improved cognitive functioning. Depression and ECT independently effect memory (Calev et al 1991).

ECT is a safe treatment associated with 2 deaths per 100 000 treatments (Royal College of Psychiatrists 1995). This compares to 0.5 deaths per 10 000 prescriptions for TCAs. This comparison may be less valid now in the era of the relatively safe SSRIs.

Does It Cause Brain Damage?

ECT does not cause brain damage. All studies to date demonstrate no damage to the brain either on investigation by CT or MRI brain scans or by post-mortem histological examination. No loss of brain cells have been demonstrated in animal studies following electroconvulsive stimulus (ECS).

Concordance/Compliance/Acceptability

ECT has a particular capacity to engender apprehension and distress in patients. A full explanation of the treatment must be given, and provision of adequate facilities to allow for safety, privacy and dignity.

MIND, the leading mental health charity in the UK, surveyed people who had undergone ECT. They report that only 14% had been given any information about it and only 9% remembered being told of adverse effects. In those treated with ECT, 43% reported that it was helpful or very helpful and 37% reported it as unhelpful or very unhelpful. MIND (1995) raised concerns in relation to regional variations in the frequency with which therapy is administered and the apparent excess of treatments administered to elderly women.

SUMMARY

Convulsive therapy was the first effective physical treatment for depression. Electroconvulsive therapy, introduced in the late 1930s in Italy, allowed for the induction of more controlled and safer seizure activity. ECT has been modified by the inclusion of general anaesthesia, with the administration of muscle relaxants from the late 1940s, which has improved safety and patient acceptability. Early trials showed high levels of efficacy, which agrees with clinical experience. The research base of earlier trials is now in question, and later trials have been limited by practical and ethical considerations. With the advent of effective antidepressant medication, the use of ECT has decreased. It is indicated in those with severe illness, treatment resistance and in specific indications such as neuro-psychological conditions, the physically ill, the elderly, pregnancy and the puerperium. This is particularly when an early response to treatment is needed. It is safe, and in the most vulnerable of patients it may be the treatment of choice. Its main role is to end an episode of depression or mania. In common with antidepressants or mood stabilisers, withdrawal of treatment without provision of prophylaxis or maintenance predicts a high rate of relapse. It is a treatment associated with high levels of antipathy in society, restricting its application. It nevertheless remains one of the central therapeutic strategies in the management of major mental health disorder.

REFERENCES

American Psychiatric Association (1990) *The Practice of Electroconvulsive Therapy: recommendations for Treatment, Training, and Privileging* American Psychiatric Press: Washington, DC

Abrams R (1994) The treatment that will not die *Psychiat Clinics of North America* **17**(3): 525–30

Abrams R et al 1983) Bilateral versus unilateral electroconvulsive therapy efficacy in melancholia *Am J Psychiat* **140**(4): 463–5

Barraclough B, Bunch J, Nelson B & Sainsbury P (1974) A hundred cases of suicide: clinical aspects *Br J Psychiat* **125**: 355–73

Barnes RC, Hussein A, Anderson DN & Powell D (1997) Maintenance electroconvulsive therapy and cognitive function *Br J Psychiat* **170**: 285–7

Barton JL, Mehta S & Snaith RP (1973) Prophylactic value of ECT in depressive illness *Acta Psychiat Scand* **49**: 386–92

Benbow SM (1995) ECT in the elderly patient. In *The ECT Handbook* The Royal College of Psychiatrists: London p 17

Bonner D & Howard R (1995) Treatment resistant depression in the elderly *Internat J Geriatric Psychiat* **10**(4): 259–64

Brandon S, Cowley P, McDonald C et al (1984) Electroconvulsive therapy: results in depressive illness from the Leicestershire trial *Br Med J* **288**: 23–5

Bridges PK, Hodgkiss AD & Malizia AL (1995) Practical management of treatment resistant affective disorders *Br J Hosp Med* **54**(10): 501–6

Buchan H, Johnstone EC, McPherson K et al (1992) Who benefits from electroconvulsive therapy? Combined results of the Leicester and Northwick Park Trials *Br J Psychiat* **160**: 355–9

Calev A, Nigal D, Shapira B, Tubi N, Chazan S, Ben-Yehuda Y, Kugelmass S & Lerer B (1991) Early and long term effects of electroconvulsive therapy and depression on memory and other cognitive functions *J Nerv Ment Dis* **179**: 526–33

Clinical Research Centre, Division of Psychiatry (1984) The Northwick Park ECT trial: Predictors of response to real and simulated ECT *Br J Psychiat* **144**: 227–37

Davis JM, Janicak PG, Sakkas P et al (1991) Electroconvulsive therapy in the treatment of the neuroleptic malignant syndrome *Convul Ther* **7**: 111–20

Dinan TG (1998) The antidepressants. In *Understanding Treatment of Mental Health Disorder* Wiley: London

Fink M (1979) *Convulsive Therapy: Theory and Practice* Raven Press: New York

Frank E, Kupfer DJ, Perel J et al (1990) Three year outcomes for maintenance therapies in recurrent depression *Arch Gen Psychiat* **47**: 1093–9

Godber C, Rosenvinge H, Wilkinson D et al (1987) Depression in old age: prognosis after ECT. *Geriat Psychiat* **2**: 19

Johns CA & Thompson JW (1995) Adjunctive treatments in schizophrenia: pharmacotherapies and electroconvulsive therapy *Schizophrenia Bull* **21**: 607–19

Johnstone EC, Deakin JFW, Lawley P et al (1980) The Northwick Park ECT trial *Lancet* **ii**: 1317–20

Kendell RE (1981) The present state of electroconvulsive therapy *Br J Psychiat* **139**: 265–83

Mann JJ & Kapur S (1994) Elucidation of biochemical basis of the antidepressant action of electroconvulsive therapy by human studies *Psychopharmacol Bull* **30**: 445–53

MRC Clinical Psychiatry Committee (1965) Clinical trial of the treatment of depressive illness. *Br Med J* **i**: 881–6

Miller LJ (1994) Use of electroconvulsive therapy during pregnancy *Hosp Comm Psychiat* **45**: 444–50

MIND (1995) *Making Sense of Treatments and Drugs: ECT* pp 4–5

Mukherjee S, Sackheim HA & Schnur DB (1994) Electroconvulsive therapy of acute manic episodes: a review of 50 years' experience [see comments]. *Am J Psychiat* **151**: 169–76

Nobler MS & Sackheim HA (1994) Refractory depression and electroconvulsive therapy. In *Refractory Depression* Wiley: Chichester pp 69–81

Pippard J (1992) Audit of electroconvulsive treatment in two national health service regions *Br J Psychiat* **160**: 621–37

Rohland BM, Carroll BT & Jacoby RG (1993) ECT in the treatment of the catatonic syndrome. *J Affect Dis* **29**: 255–61

Royal College of Psychiatrists (1995) *The ECT Handbook* (ed CP Freeman) p 4

Sackheim HA (1994) Continuation therapy following ECT: directions for future research *Psychopharmacol Bull* **30**: 501–21

Scott AI & Whalley LJ (1993) The onset and rate of the antidepressant effect of elctroconvulsive therapy. A neglected area of research [see comments] *Br J Psychiat* **162**: 725–32.

Weiner RD, Rodgers HJ, Davidson JRT & Squire LR (1986) Effects of stimulus parameters on cognitive side effects *Ann NY Acad Sci* **462**

Weschler H, Grosser GH & Greenblatt M (1965) Research evaluating antidepressant medications on hospitalised mental patients: a survey of published reports during a five year period *J Nerv Ment Dis* **141**: 231–9

CHAPTER 8

Prophylaxis of Affective Disorders

David Healy and Tom McMonagle

University of Wales

INTRODUCTION

This chapter will cover one of the most contentious areas in psychiatry. The idea that people should stay on treatment for long periods of time, even for life, is problematic. This is particularly so in depression, which is perceived by some as 'not such a serious disorder' or a disorder which should be 'sorted out by talking'.

The chapter covers a group of drug treatments once termed *mood stabilisers*. This term is falling out of use and our focus will be more on what it is hoped treatment will do, rather than on the intrinsic properties of the drugs. There will be no reference to possible mechanisms of action of the various drugs, as there is no consensus on these issues. The reader will also need to look elsewhere for details of dosages and side-effects (see Healy 1997a). The plan of the chapter is to look at lithium, the antidepressants and the anticonvulsants to see how the notion of mood prophylaxis emerged. An effort will be made to integrate pharmaco-therapeutic and behavioural approaches and to say something about issues of compliance.

Understanding Psychiatric Treatment. Edited by G. O'Mahony and J.V. Lucey.

LITHIUM

In 1952 Mogens Schou started what was probably the first randomised placebo-controlled trial in psychiatry using lithium in patients with mania (Schou et al 1954). Three groups of patients entered the study. One group had chronic mania, a second had episodic mania, and were currently manic, and the third consisted of one person who regularly cycled rapidly between manic and depressive episodes. This latter subject entered the study when manic and improved significantly. It was noted that not only had his mania improved but he had stopped cycling between manic and depressive episodes.

Nothing more of that observation was made until 1959 when PC Baastrup from Copenhagen and Tobias Hartigan from Canterbury independently contacted Schou and raised the possibility that lithium might have a prophylactic action against further depressive or manic episodes. This was based on observations that both had made in their clinical practice (Johnson 1984). Part of the reason to claim a prophylactic action was that patients with manic-depressive illnesses appeared to be having fewer depressive episodes while on lithium. This was significant because the antidepressant effects of lithium were unconvincing and the implication was that lithium was warding off further episodes rather than treating a current episode. Schou and Baastrup subsequently followed the clinical course of manic depressive illness in a large number of subjects who had had regular episodes in previous years. Subjects who stayed on lithium had fewer episodes than previously, while those who halted treatment relapsed quickly. This was an open study but it led them to claims that lithium appeared to have a prophylactic action in mood disorders (Baastrup and Schou 1967).

This claim triggered a controversy. Professor Michael Shepherd and others, questioned the proposition. The sceptics had a number of arguments. One was the possibility that lithium prophylaxis might be mediated by a psychological mechanism. Alternatively the natural course of the illness might be giving the impression that things had improved. The argument was that all the subjects entered the study because they had experienced a recent severe episode of illness and, in the natural course of illness, these bad periods should be followed by good periods. In response to the argument that subjects who came off lithium appeared to relapse, they suggested this might be evidence of a lithium withdrawal syndrome. Shepherd began one of the major controversies in psychopharmacology, setting out the questions that any claim for a prophylactic action by a treatment must address (Blackwell and Shepherd 1968; Shepherd and Healy 1998).

In casting these doubts on the prophylactic effects of lithium, Shepherd and his colleagues opened a debate that was vigorously fought on both sides. Schou and others subsequently demonstrated that the course of affective illness is such that the assumptions he and Baastrup had made about lithium's prophylactic effects were justified. It appears that in a manic depressive illness, episodes come with increasing frequency over the years. It is improbable that, if there are fewer episodes following a prophylactic agent such as lithium, this is explained by fluctuations in the natural course of the illness. In response to claims that the discontinuation of lithium might lead to mania, as part of a withdrawal effect, Schou argued that the evidence was inadequate (Schou 1993). To demonstrate this effect, discontinuation should be initiated by the therapist, not the patient. If the patient stops treatment this is likely, in some cases, to be secondary to mood elevation (Schou 1997; Schou and Healy 1998).

A series of randomised trials comparing placebo and lithium were initiated. A further argument from Shepherd had been that patients were being selected for a good response. There are ethical difficulties with trials in this area. It is one thing to randomise mildly depressed patients to placebo for a few weeks, but is it justifiable to do so for a more seriously ill group for periods of over a year? Despite these difficulties a series of trials were run and these showed that individuals taking lithium had a significantly lower rate of relapse compared with those taking placebo (Baastrup et al 1970; Coppen et al 1971).

Since then a number of naturalistic studies have followed up the original randomised control studies demonstrating that subjects who take lithium show significant benefits other than a reduction in affective episodes leading to hospitalisation. Rates of suicide among manic depressive subjects are seven to eight times those of the general population. While on lithium these rates fall to the level of the general population, but they rise again in subjects who discontinue their lithium (Coppen and Healy 1996; Schou 1997).

These trials focused on subjects with bipolar disorders, but other trials examined lithium use in recurrent unipolar depression. There is less agreement about the outcome of such studies. Some evidence points to the efficacy of lithium in preventing recurrence of unipolar depressions but at present the preferred option appears to be continued use of antidepressants (Schou 1997; Kupfer and Frank 1997). Is this because of fewer side-effects and greater ease of administration, or because the antidepressants in addition to being antidepressant in acute episodes are also prophylactic? One of the problems with electroconvulsive therapy is that although it is a potent treatment in acute episodes and is an antidepressant, responses appear to be followed in a high proportion of relapses in the short term.

ANTIDEPRESSANTS

When the antidepressants were originally given, it was clear that a number of subjects needed to remain on them for considerable periods of time, if not indefinitely. As early as 1958, Roland Kuhn reported that he had subjects who were on imipramine treatment for two years (Kuhn 1958; Healy 1997b). Some subjects got well quickly and in this case it was possible to discontinue treatment, but in others Kuhn felt treatment should be continued on a symptomatic basis. The need to continue treatment indefinitely in some patients led to a proposal as early as 1959 that imipramine might be addictive, on the basis that discontinuing it led to relapse.

During the 1960s, it was thought that antidepressant treatment did not need to be lengthy. This was influenced by recent introduction of randomised clinical trials as part of the registration process for psychotropic compounds. These trials were conducted because regulatory bodies, such as the Food & Drug Administration in the USA, required proof of efficacy of a compound before they would license it. Proof that a drug *gets* patients well is different to proof that the drugs *keep them well* for lengthy periods of time. In order to demonstrate efficacy, clinical trial protocols commonly involved the comparison of an antidepressant with another antidepressant or with placebo over a trial period that only lasted 4–6 weeks. This was sufficient time to register the fact that the drug 'worked' but not sufficient time to establish whether it was useful in the longer term. Under the influence of such trials, an impression arose that treatment with an antidepressant was not different to treatment with an antibiotic. According to this view, a short course of treatment might be effective, regardless of behavioural measures and independent of the patient's psychosocial milieu.

Recently it has been established that this is not the case. Studies were conducted during the 1970s and 1980s looking at the effects of continued treatment with antidepressants, following initial therapeutic response. It became clear that treatment for 6 or 12 months following initial recovery of depressive episodes significantly reduced relapse rates (Glen, Johnston and Shepherd 1984). The rates of relapse on placebo in the year following treatment have been between 50 and 80%. The rates with continued imipramine or amitriptyline treatment have been 30% or less (Healy 1997b).

The most influential studies on relapse rates come from Pittsburgh and have been conducted by David Kupfer, Ellen Frank and colleagues. Kupfer and Frank randomised patients with recurrent episodes of depression to maintenance treatment with interpersonal therapy (IPT), imipramine, or placebo, for three and subsequently five years (Frank et al 1990). Over the initial three-year period, treatment with either full-dose imipramine or IPT significantly reduced rates of relapse, while placebo relapse rates were substantial. For those not taking medication, continued IPT significantly increased survival time.

There are widely accepted distinctions between recurrences and relapses (Frank et al 1991). When a patient initially responds to an antidepressant the underlying disorder may not necessarily have resolved. In some cases they may have recovered; but in more severe cases, or in those liable to recurrence, there is another possibility. Treatment can relieve some symptoms but the underlying problem remains masked. The patient has not truly recovered, but is rather in a remission. Discontinuation of treatment in such circumstances will lead to a re-emergence of the initial problem – a relapse. In contrast, a recurrence is an episode of depression that occurs some time after recovery and discontinuation of treatment; it has all the hallmarks of a new episode rather than the re-emergence of a previous episode. Within this framework, antidepressants have different actions. One is that they cure an episode of depression. Another is that they treat a current episode symptomatically until it resolves itself – they can induce a remission. A third possibility is that they might bring about a recovery additionally reducing the liability to recurrences.

Emerging findings from different classes of antidepressants may be pertinent. The development of the selective serotonin (5HT) re-uptake inhibitors (SSRIs: citalopram, fluoxetine, fluvoxamine, paroxetine and sertraline) indicated that an action on the 5HT serotonergic system could be an antidepressant principle. It was hoped that these treatments might be a more specific cure for depression – a so-called *magic bullet*. However, studies through the 1980s suggested that the SSRIs were less potent in treating severely depressed hospitalised patients than were older tricyclic antidepressants active on both noradrenergic and serotonergic systems (DUAG 1990; Bech and Healy 1998). The implication of this is that the SSRIs are an antidepressant principle rather than a specific treatment. An antidepressant principle is anything that will contribute to any extent over and above the effects of a placebo to the amelioration of some aspects of a depressive disorder (Healy and McMonagle 1977). Action on the noradrenergic system might also offer an antidepressant principle; similarly, it is suggested that antidepressants selected exclusively for the noradrenergic system (desipramine and maprotiline) are less effective than drugs with both noradrenergic and serotonergic activity. What are these two groups of drugs doing that is useful in depression, but which falls short of a specific cure for it?

One possibility is that drugs active on the noradrenergic system do something different to drugs active on the serotonergic system. What might this be? There has for some time been a tradition that drugs, such as desipramine, that are active on catecholamine systems are more motor activating than drugs active on the indoleamine serotonin system. When the physiological systems in the brain – for which noradrenaline and serotonin are the primary neurotransmitters – were first mapped out, these distinctions were expressed in terms of ergotrophic (work/arousal) systems and a trophotrophic (vegetative) system respectively. With the discovery of neurotransmitters it was clear that noradrenaline was the principal neurotransmitter in the work/arousal ergotrophic systems and serotonin in the vegetative trophotrophic system. If this is valid one possibility is that an action on noradrenaline systems might be more effective in breaking the autonomy of a depressive episode by their activating effects, while an action on the serotonin system might do something else.

A recent study by Bech and colleagues in Denmark took a severely depressed group of patients and randomised them to ECT and placebo, ECT and imipramine or ECT and paroxetine. Subjects on ECT and imipramine got better marginally quicker than the other groups. Relapse rates were highest in those maintained on placebo. They were significantly lower in those treated with paroxetine compared with those maintained on imipramine. This suggests that an action on the 5HT system might be more *prophylactic* than an action on the noradrenergic system or prophylactic in a way that activity on the noradrenergic system is not (Lauritzen et al 1996). ECT, or drugs active on numbers of transmitter systems in contrast seem better able to treat a severe depressive episode.

Further studies of the sequence of events and appearance of symptoms during relapse revealed that subjects became mildly irritable and withdrew socially prior to developing poor sleep and poor appetite, ultimately going on to ideas of guilt and thoughts of suicide (Bech and Healy 1997). In terms of activity of the 5HT system, there is a considerable amount of evidence to suggest that these agents are anxiolytic in some way and one possibility is that they modulate irritability (Van Praag 1993). It is possible therefore that an anti-irritability/anti-nervousness action mediated through the serotonin system might forestall social withdrawal and prevent relapse.

It may be that lithium acts in a similar way to the SSRIs. It is also less effective in severe depression and it, too, has an anti-irritability action beneficial in the management of aggression. There remains dispute about the relative merits of antidepressants, including the SSRIs and lithium in the management of recurrent unipolar depressions. There is evidence that lithium is useful (Prien et al 1984; Schou 1997) but antidepressants are probably favoured over lithium, in part for reasons of convenience (Kupfer and Frank 1997).

ANTICONVULSANTS

The anticonvulsants, carbamazepine and sodium valproate, appear to have some prophylactic potential for mood disorders, so much so that most newly developed anticonvulsants, such as lamotrigine, are now also being assessed for possible prophylactic activity.

Carbamazepine

In 1949, imipramine was derived from an immino-dibenzyl nucleus which was synthesised in 1898. It was first used in 1955. Carbamazepine is a related drug, developed from the same nucleus, which was first synthesised in 1957 (Healy 1997b). This compound had more potent anti-epileptic properties than other tricyclic compounds and during the 1980s became a drug of first choice for convulsive disorders. In the course of its use in epilepsy, it was reported by Pierre Lambert, as early as 1965, to have 'mood-stabilising' properties, and subsequent studies in Japan confirmed this. In the 1980s, carbamazepine came into widespread use in the management of bipolar affective disorders, although no large-scale randomised trials were ever undertaken to confirm its efficacy. It appears to have some efficacy in the management of mania, but again this has not been established as clearly as it has for lithium.

Given that carbamazepine is a tricyclic agent with marked structural similarities to imipramine, its efficacy is not surprising. At present, there are few indications as to how it works. It seems to have an anti-irritability effect and it has been used in the management of a disorder termed 'episodic dyscontrol syndrome'. It is also useful in recurrent disorders such as trigeminal neuralgia. Carbamazepine has a niche in patients who are unresponsive to lithium, or unable to tolerate its side-effects, as well as in patients who have atypical dysphoric affective disorders or schizo-affective disorders. In general, the closer the patient is to manic-depressive disorder – with clear endogenous depressions and manias characterised by grandiose and euphoric moods – the more the patient is likely to respond to lithium; whereas the more complicated and atypical the picture, the greater the likelihood that the patient will respond to carbamazepine. The only direct comparison between lithium and carbamazepine to date suggests that lithium is effective in more patients than is carbamazepine (Greil et al forthcoming).

Valproic Acid (Sodium Valproate)

Valproic Acid is a branched fatty acid which was first synthesised in 1882. It was re-discovered in the 1940s in war-time Germany as part of a programme to supplement the chronic shortage of petrol and as a possible butter substitute. Its nutritional value was poor but it appeared relatively safe (Meijer, Meinardi and Binnie 1983). Valproic acid first came into use as an anticonvulsant almost by accident. In the early 1960s it was used as an oil base into which bismuth was instilled for the treatment of tonsillitis. During these experiments it produced striking muscle relaxation which led to further investigation, and its anti-epileptic properties were discovered in 1962.

Again, the possible prophylactic effects of valproic acid on mood disorders were first proposed by Pierre Lambert. Subsequent studies have found it to be an effective anti-manic agent having a mood-stabilising action in a proportion of people who are manic depressive (Balfour and Bryson 1994; Healy 1997a). In general, the populations that are unresponsive to lithium, for whom carbamazepine might be considered, are the group who are most likely to respond to valproate. It has efficacy for both unipolar and bipolar depressions but its place in therapy is as yet not fully established. At present there is no evidence that it is superior to either lithium or carbamazepine for manic-depressive disorder. Lithium is still the first choice treatment.

BEHAVIOURAL APPROACHES TO PROPHYLAXIS

As noted above, one of the most influential studies of prophylaxis compared imipramine to interpersonal therapy and found that both were able to ward off the emergence of further episodes, whether relapses or recurrences (Frank et al 1990). Interpersonal therapy emerged in the mid-1970s when it was shown to have effects both in the acute treatment of depression but also in enhancing social functioning during the maintenance treatment of depression following an acute episode. The strategy behind IPT is to engage the individual in tackling troublesome areas of interpersonal functioning they may have. Based on the analysis of antidepressant principles above it can be proposed that this type of action might counteract the withdrawal that Bech and colleagues found occurs in the early stages of an effective episode.

Frank and colleagues have gone further and developed an Interpersonal and Social Rhythm Therapy (Frank et al 1994), which incorporates behavioural hygiene principles. This was developed in part because of evidence of circadian system dysfunction in affective disorders. Of interest here are findings from Adeniran and colleagues (1996) who have shown that circadian rhythm disruption of the kind that occurs in subjects taking on nightwork leads to an increase in sensitivity to criticism from significant others and irritability as well as most of the symptoms of depression such as disturbed sleep, appetite, concentration and interest.

The other non-pharmacotherapeutic approach to affective disorders at present is cognitive therapy (CT). Treatment studies have shown it has some efficacy in the treatment of mild to moderate depressive episodes. There has only been one study (the NIMH collaborative treatment study) in which CT was compared to imipramine, IPT and clinical management alone (a package of sensible advice and behavioural hygiene principles). In this the data suggested that the more severe the depressive episode the more likely imipramine and IPT were to be effective compared to cognitive therapy or clinical management (Elkin et al 1989). In addition to its acute effects in depression, there have been claims that cognitive therapy might reduce rates of relapse. In the NIMH study, there was a lower rate of relapse in those who had responded to cognitive therapy compared with those responding to IPT or imipramine but the lowest relapse rates were in those responding to clinical management alone. This illustrates the hazards of prophylactic studies. Arguably what has happened here is that those who responded to cognitive therapy or clinical management (placebo) were individuals who were less likely to relapse anyway and claiming that the therapy they had had anything to do with making them less likely to relapse is problematic.

What is there about cognitive therapy that might be prophylactic against a relapse? There are a number of components to CT as outlined in treatment manuals. These include a cognitive element which aims at tackling errors in logic that the subject is making, a further exploratory component that aims at unearthing depressive complexes the individual may harbour and finally a behavioural activation component which involves mobilisation of the subject through homework exercises and activity schedules. To date there has been little systematic investigation of the differential effectiveness of each of these components apart from one study by Jacobsen and colleagues (1996) which found all three components to be equally effective. It remains possible therefore that IPT and CT operate through similar mechanisms – problem solving, especially in the interpersonal domain, and behaviour scheduling.

There is one group of recurrent depressions in particular where non-pharmacotherapeutic approaches appear to have some efficacy; these are the 'seasonal' depressions. There is some doubt that these are seasonal in the sense of being caused by changes in the photoperiod but there is no doubt that they are recurrent. At present all approaches toward their management, whether the use of light therapies in the morning, or the scheduling of early morning exercise, rather notably involve programmes of behavioural activation and efforts to counter tendencies to social withdrawal.

PREDICTORS OF RELAPSE

There are a number of predictors of depressive episodes. These include the levels of depressive symptoms premorbidly (Horwath et al 1992), the severity and frequency of any previous episodes, levels of neuroticism (Angst 1992) and sensitivity to interpersonal criticism (Hooley et al 1986; Adeniran et al 1996).

The significance of high levels of pre-existing depressive symptoms as a predictor of subsequent relapse is that it implies that some people who recover from a depressive episode do not make a full recovery and are left with a diminution of self-esteem or other 'scaring' afterwards. Findings such as this fit with the notions outlined by Frank above. In these cases, treatment whether an antidepressant or a psychotherapy can be seen as having induced an incomplete remission rather than a recovery. Individuals in this state arguably are the ones to whom therapeutic attentions should be addressed. In individuals who remain symptomatic despite vigorous antidepressant treatment the suspicion must be that there are compounding psychological factors that should be addressed. Addressing personality factors such as levels of neuroticism, however, is no easy matter.

One of the best known predictors of a depressive episode of any kind is life events. The environmental dislocations that they bring about may precipitate a variety of affective reactions, including melancholias and manias. A note of caution needs to be sounded here in that in the course of the first prophylactic study carried out by Baastrup and Schou, the authors found that almost all the subjects who relapsed blamed their fresh episode on concurrent stressors. Relapses, however, almost uniformly came from the placebo rather than the lithium group, which suggests that these setbacks owed more to the 'endogenous rhythm of the manic-depressive illness' than to the consequences of environmental disturbances (Schou 1997a). An alternative might be that individuals subject to affective disorders are more vulnerable to the disrupting effects of life events than normal and that treatment attenuates this vulnerability.

PROPHYLAXIS OR NOT?

The first point to be made here is that the majority of the studies referred to above have been on severely depressed hospitalised populations. These are not representative of the majority of depressive episodes. The simple recurrence of an episode does not necessarily imply that prophylaxis should be considered.

On the other hand once a depressive disorder has become severe enough to warrant hospitalisation and once it has also shown a tendency to recurrence, the risks of suicide rise substantially and there is a good evidence that rates of hospitalisation and of suicide can be significantly reduced by treatment aimed at prophylaxis.

One of the problems of long-term treatment is compliance. This is a neglected topic in mental health research. To date there are no clear indications of how compliance can be reliably optimised. It is perhaps worth bearing in mind, however, that compliance is never simply a matter of adhering to a regime of pills, be they lithium or SSRIs. Owing to the current regulation of psychopharmaceuticals, individuals who want treatments can only access them through medical prescribers. Failures of compliance therefore are as likely to reflect failures in the therapeutic skills of the prescriber or in their basic capacities to relate to others as they are to stem from any 'lack of insight' on the part of the taker of the medications.

A second problem is that at present the pharmaceutical industry are better placed to establish evidence of prophylactic efficacy than are any other group in the mental health arena. This being so, prescribers should be aware that the absence of evidence of efficacy for programmes of behaviour scheduling and problem solving, in particular interpersonal problem solving, is not evidence of an absence of efficacy. There is indeed suggestive evidence that such approaches should be built into any treatment packages aimed at reducing the likelihood of relapse in either unipolar or bipolar affective disorders.

REFERENCES

Adeniran R, Healy D, Sharp H, Williams JMG, Minors D & Waterhouse JM (1996) Interpersonal sensitivity predicts depressive symptom response to the circadian rhythm disruption of nightwork *Psychol Med* **26**: 1211–21

Angst J (1992) How recurrent and predictable is depressive disorder. In S Montgomery & F Rouillon (eds) *Long-term Treatment of Depression* Wiley: Chichester pp 1–14

Baastrup PC &Schou M (1967) Lithium as a prophylactic agent: its effects against recurrent depressions and manic-depressive psychosis *Arch Gen Psychiat* **16**: 162–72

Baastrup PC, Poulsen JC, Schou M, Thomsen K & Amdisen A (1970) Prophylactic lithium: double-blind discontinuation in manic-depressive and recurrent depressive disorders *Lancet* **ll**: 326–30

Balfour JA & Bryson HM (1994) Valproic acid: a review of its pharmacology and therapeutic potential in indications other than epilepsy. *CNS Drugs* **2**: 144–73

Bech P & Healy D (1998) Measurement and organisation in psychopharmacology. In D Healy (ed) *The Psychopharmacologists* vol 2 Chapman & Hall: London

Blackwell B & Shepherd M (1968) Prophylactic lithium: another therapeutic myth. A consideration of the evidence *Lancet* **2**: 968–70

Coppen A, Noguera R, Bailey J, Burns BH, Swami MS, Hare EH, Gardner R & Maggs R (1971) Prophylactic lithium in affective disorders. Controlled trial *Lancet* **1**: 275–79

Coppen A & Healy D (1996) Biological psychiatry in the United Kingdom. In D Healy (ed) *The Psychopharmacologists* vol 1 Chapman & Hall: London pp 265–86

Danish Universities Antidepressant Group (DUAG) (1990) Paroxetine. A selective serotonin reuptake inhibitor showing better tolerance but weaker antidepressant effect than clomipramine in a controlled multicenter study *J Affect Dis* **18**: 289–99

Elkin I, Shea TM, Watkins JT, Imber SD, Sotsky SM, Collins JF, Glass DR, Pilkonis PA, Leber WR, Docherty JP, Fiester SJ & Parloff MB (1989) NIMH treatment of depression collaborative research programme: general effectiveness of treatments *Arch Gen Psychiat* **46**: 971–82

Frank E, Kupfer D, Perel JM, Cornes C, Jarrett DB, Mallinger AG, Thase ME, McEachran AB & Grochocinski VJ (1990) Three year outcomes for maintenance therapies in recurrent depression *Arch Gen Psychiat* **47**: 1093–99

Frank E, Prien RF, Jarrett RB et al (1991) Conceptualisation and rationale for consensus definitions of terms in major depressive disorder: remission, recovery, relapse and recurrence *Arch Gen Psychiat* **48**: 851–5

Frank E, Kupfer DJ, Ehlers C, Monk TH, Cornes C, Carter S & Frankel D (1994) Interpersonal and social rhythm therapy *Behav Ther* **17**: 143–49

Glen AIM, Johnson AL & Shepherd M (1984) Continuation therapy with lithium and amitriptyline in unipolar depressive illness: a randomised double-blind controlled trial *Psychol Med* **14**: 37–50

Healy D (1997a) *Psychiatric Drugs Explained* Mosby Yearbooks Ltd: London

Healy D (1997b) *The Antidepressant Era* Harvard University Press: Cambridge, MA

Healy D & McMonagle T (1997) The enhancement of social functioning as a therapeutic principle in the management of depression *J Psychopharmacology* **11**, s25–32

Hooley JM, Orley J & Teasdale JD (1986) Levels of expressed emotion and relapse in depressed patients *Br J Psychiat* **148**: 642–47

Horwath E, Johnson J, Klerman GL & Weissman MM (1992) Depressive symptoms as relative and attributable risk factors for first onset-major depression *Arch Gen Psychiat* **49**: 817–23

Jacobson NS, Dobson KS, Truax PA, Addis ME, Koerner K, Gollan JK, Gortner E & Prince SE (1996) A component analysis of cognitive behavior therapy for depression *J Consult Clin Psychol* **64**: 295–304

Johnson FN (1984) *The History of Lithium Therapy* Macmillan: London

Klerman GL, Weissman MM, Rounsaville BJ & Chevron ES (1984) *Interpersonal Therapy of Depression* Basic Books: New York

Kuhn R (1958) The treatment of depressive states with G22355 (imipramine hydrochloride) *Am J Psychiat* **115**: 459–64

Kupfer D & Frank E (1997) Forty years of lithium treatment *Arch Gen Psychiat* **54**: 14–15

Lauritzen L, Odgaard K, Clemmesen L, Lunde M, Orstrom J, Black C & Bech P (1996) Relapse prevention by means of paroxetine in ECT-treated patients with major depression: a comparison with imipramine and placebo in medium-term continuation therapy *Acta Psychiat Scand* **94**: 241–51

Meijer JWA, Meinardi H & Binnie CD (1983) The development of anti-epileptic drugs. In MJ Parnham & J Bruinvels (eds) *Discoveries in Pharmacology* Elsevier: London pp 447–78

Prien RF, Kupfer DJ, Mansky PA, Small JG, Tuason VB, Voss CB & Johnson WE (1984) Drug therapy in the prevention of recurrences in unipolar and bipolar affective disorders *Arch Gen Psychiat* **41**: 1096–104

Schou M, Juel-Nielsen N, Stromgren E & Voldby H (1954) The treatment of manic psychoses by the administration of lithium salts *J Neurolog Neurosurg Psychiat* **17**: 250–60

Schou M (1993) Is there a lithium withdrawal syndrome? An examination of the evidence *Br J Psychiat* **163**: 514–8

Schou M (1997) Forty years of lithium treatment *Arch Gen Psychiat* **54**: 9–13

Schou M & Healy D (1998) Lithium. In D Healy (ed) *The Psychopharmacologists* vol 2 Chapman & Hall: London

Shepherd M & Healy D (1998) Specific and non-specific effects in psychopharmacology. In D Healy (ed) *The Psychopharmacologists* vol 2 Chapman & Hall: London

Van Praag M (1993) *'Make-Believes' in Psychiatry or The Perils of Progress* Brunner-Mazel: New York

CHAPTER 9

Antipsychotic Treatment of Patients with Schizophrenia

Robert W. Kerwin

Institute of Psychiatry, London

Ann Mortimer

North Wales Hospital, Clwyd

and

Kevin Lynch

Institute of Psychiatry, London

INTRODUCTION

There are a variety of disorders collectively described as the group of schizophrenias. Their phenomenology and symptom profile is heterogeneous, with a variety of social, neuropsychological, physiological and structural correlates (Andreason et al 1995). Current classification is descriptive rather than based on conceptual or aetiological grounds. Treatment strategies aim at ameliorating symptoms and modifying the course and outcome of illness. There is no cure; there are physical, psychological and social interventions. The introduction of the antipsychotic medications, the neuroleptics,

Understanding Psychiatric Treatment. Edited by G. O'Mahony and J.V. Lucey.

from the 1950s, contributed to the transfer of management from institutional care to the community.

DEVELOPMENT

The first neuroleptic, chlorpromazine, was synthesised in 1950. It was developed as one of a number of antihistamine compounds being investigated at the time. Laborit, a French anaesthetist, is credited with first noting that promethazine, a phenothiazine antihistamine, possessed effects as a calming agent during anaesthesia. Based upon his initial observations and suggestions to the psychiatric community, chlorpromazine was introduced in France, and initially used in combination with barbiturates. Jean Delay and Pierre Deniker first described the use of the drug in psychiatric practice as a separate treatment. Deniker suggested the name 'neuroleptic' in 1955 in distinction to the earlier term 'psycholeptic' used for sedative or hypnotic drugs which solely reduced psychological tension. The new compound appeared to have effects both mental and neurological. The demonstration of therapeutic benefit led to a series of developments with the synthesis of a range of neuroleptic compounds. The common pharmacological action of these agents was an effect upon the dopaminergic neurotransmitter, with blockade of central dopamine receptors. All effective neuroleptics show some affinity for the dopamine (D2) receptor site (Livingston 1994; Healy 1991). With growing knowledge of neuroleptic pharmacology came an awareness that other neurotransmitters may be targeted by effective antipsychotic medication, such as the serotonergic (5HT) system. Early acceptance of the benefits of treatment with dopamine antagonists is now tempered by experience of the adverse effects of medication.

RISKS OF TRADITIONAL NEUROLEPTICS

The traditional neuroleptics are associated with neuroendocrine, autonomic and motor system side-effects, in addition to influencing a range of neurotransmitter receptors: dopaminergic, adrenergic, cholinergic, histaminergic and serotonergic. As well as objective biological effects, there is the subjective response of users, the so-called *ataritic* state of induced calmness or indifference. For some this is an unpleasant detachment or deadening of experiences. Most neuroleptics induce weight gain and through elevation of prolactin levels may stimulate galactorrhoea. They induce hypotension, cardiac arrhythmias and interfere with sexual function. The most visible and disabling affects are those on motor function involving the extrapyramidal system.

Movement Disorders/ExtraPyramidal Side-Effects (EPSE)

In patients treated with neuroleptics, 5% experience acute dystonia with adoption of distorted posture or grimacing; 40% experience drug-induced Parkinsonism, with rigidity, poverty of movement and tremor, commonly of bilateral distribution; 20% develop akathisia – an experience of objective restlessness, accompanied by subjective feelings of tension; and 30% develop dyskinesia, the most severe of which is tardive dyskinesia (Stahl and Wets 1988). The involvement of dopamine blockade in these disorders is crucial. Acute dystonia and Parkinsonism respond to anticholinergic medication. Their significance may largely be that the presence of early EPSE acts as a marker for later disabling movement disorder. The realisation that the onset of disabling movement disorder is cumulative, with its highest expression in elderly patients, makes an exploration of novel neuroleptics and reappraisal of prescribing practices more urgent. A prospective study of risk of tardive dyskinesia in older patients, studying 226 subjects with a mean age 66 years on low dose treatment (mean 150 mg chlorpromazine equivalents per day), showed a cumulative incidence of tardive dyskinesia of 26% at one year, 52% at two years and 60% at three years. This compared to younger patients, showing 5% at one year, 19% at four years and 26% at six years (Jeste et al 1995). Associated risk factors included female sex, smoking, affective illness, diabetes mellitus, substance misuse and African racial origin.

Neuroleptic Malignant Syndrome

This is a relatively rare, potentially fatal, idiosyncratic reaction to neuroleptic medication. It consists of pyrexia, autonomic nervous system instability, muscular rigidity and altered level of consciousness. There are widely differing estimates of its incidence, depending on the diagnostic criteria used and the level of suspicion. Its likely incidence is 0.2% of neuroleptic users (Kohen and Bristow 1996). It is most likely to occur in the first two weeks after commencing or withdrawing neuroleptic treatment, although it may occur at other times. With current supportive management, fatality is now rare.

Cognitive Function

A review by King (1990) suggests that traditional neuroleptics result in impairment of psychomotor function and sustained attention, but higher cognitive functions remain unaffected. Studies show adverse effects, neutral effects and beneficial effects. The majority indicate an overall improvement in cognitive function and attention in parallel with clinical recovery.

Seizure Threshold

Neuroleptic drugs lower the seizure threshold, increasing vulnerability to epileptic discharges. This complicates their use in epileptic subjects.

WHEN SHOULD ATYPICAL NEUROLEPTICS BE USED?

The treatment of seriously ill patients with schizophrenia involves management of those who have failed to respond promptly to early interventions with antipsychotic medication, remaining behaviourally or symptomatically disturbed.

In severe forms of schizophrenia, it is important that an effective therapy is introduced as early as possible. Conventional neuroleptics share the property of central dopamine receptor blockade. Where resistance to these antipsychotics is exhibited, clozapine, an atypical agent, has proven efficacy. It is also associated with fewer extrapyramidal movement disorder side-effects than the conventional neuroleptics. Its use has, however, been limited by concerns regarding the possibility of haematological events such as agranulocytosis.

The decision to introduce newer antipsychotics is dependent on the loosely defined concept of a *difficult to treat* patient. A reasonable definition of treatment resistance might comment on the lack of improvement after six weeks or more, of at least two conventional oral neuroleptics, of different classes, at appropriate therapeutic doses. This is despite the fact that there is no pharmacological rationale for trying a second conventional agent after the failure of a first.

It may be advantageous to reduce the time spent treating patients with conventional agents when response is clearly inadequate. Instead, attention should be paid to trials of adjunctive agents or neuroleptics with atypical pharmacological actions. In the presence of a continued suboptimal clinical response, there is a need for early introduction of a drug with proven efficacy in treatment-resistant schizophrenia. Presently, clozapine alone meets this description, although newer drugs like olanzapine, sertindole, quetiapine and ziprasidone may ultimately fulfil this role.

Positive and Negative Features

Conventional neuroleptics are most effective against the positive symptoms of schizophrenia, such as delusions and hallucinations. They have less effect against negative symptoms such as emotional and social withdrawal, and reduction in activity levels. Until clozapine was shown to be more effective than conventional neuroleptics in treatment-resistant schizophrenia (Kane et al 1988), the approach to the management of this group involved switching from one neuroleptic to another of a different chemical structure. As conventional neuroleptics act predominantly at the dopamine (D2) receptor, it is not surprising that this approach was, in many cases, ineffective. By contrast, it is apparent that clozapine has a different neuropharmacological action and is the only drug with proven efficacy in this treatment group.

TREATMENT-RESISTANT SCHIZOPHRENIA

The incidence of treatment-resistant schizophrenia has been described as between 10 and 25% (Davis 1980; Lieberman et al 1991). One author gives somewhat higher figures, reporting 30% of schizophrenic patients as non-responders, and another 30–40% as partial responders (Lewander 1992). Clearly there exists a spectrum of response to neuroleptics and, therefore, treatment resistance does not equate with a total lack of response. During the 1980s an international study group attempted to clarify the concept of treatment resistance (Brenner and Merlo 1995). They established a seven-level rating scale, ranging from clinical remission at level one, to severe refractory disease at level seven. The operational diagnosis described by these authors appears unfeasible for use in clinical practice, and a number of other authors have offered more pragmatic definitions of treatment resistance (Table 9.1).

APPROACHES TO MANAGING DIFFICULT-TO-TREAT SCHIZOPHRENIA

It is important in the first instance to ensure that lack of response to first choice neuroleptics is not a result of non-compliance. It has been suggested that 40–65% of out-patients will stop their regular antipsychotic medication within six weeks (Johnson 1988). As a result, many patients may be assessed as poor responders when they are in fact being under-treated. Sometimes problems with compliance may be

Table 9.1 Definitions of treatment-resistant schizophrenia

Authors	Definition
Kane et al (1988)	No sufficient improvement after treatment with three neuroleptics of different classes (1000 mg chlorpromazine equivalent) for six weeks No episode of complete symptomatic remission during last five years
Meltzer et al (1989)	Failure to respond after treatment with at least two different neuroleptics from different classes (800 mg chlorpromazine equivalent) used for a minimum of four weeks
Keefe et al (1991)	No sufficient improvement after neuroleptic treatment (40 mg haloperidol equivalent) during six weeks
Huckle and Palia (1993)	Persistence of positive symptoms after at least three different neuroleptics from at least two classes (600 mg chlorpromazine equivalent) for minimum of four weeks while ensuring adequate compliance

addressed with intramuscular injectable depot preparations, although it should be noted that poor compliance is frequently a result of intolerance, and in particular extrapyramidal movement disorders. In the absence of antipsychotic effect from one neuroleptic drug, it is common practice to switch to another of a different chemical structure. This is based on the rationale that different classes of drug will have a different neuropharmacological mechanisms of action. Improved understanding of neuroreceptor activity indicates that all conventional antipsychotic agents occupy the dopamine D2 receptors (Seeman 1992) and, the rationale for using another typical neuroleptic may be incorrect. Earlier clinical studies are consistent with this in that none of the conventional neuroleptics has been shown to be superior to any other in terms of its clinical efficacy (Hollister et al 1974). There may, however, be a stronger argument for switching neuroleptics as a result of intolerance to any one drug.

Another approach has been to increase dosage of the neuroleptic to a maximum tolerated dose, although a number of controlled trials have not suggested any advantage in giving high doses of conventional neuroleptics (Hirsch 1986). A recent randomised double-blind clinical trial examined 87 hospitalised patients with schizophrenia (Rifkin et al 1991). In this study, there was no difference between patients who failed to respond, whether they received a four-week course of standard antipsychotic (fluphenazine 20 mg per day), or another four weeks of therapy with the same treatment, or a higher dose, or a different medication (haloperidol up to 80 mg per day). However, the same author suggests that if patients do not respond well to doses of the order of 10–20 mg per day of haloperidol, then doses of up to 40–60 mg per day should be tried for up to six weeks. This view is supported in a review of the treatment of neuroleptic non-responsive patients by Meltzer (1992).

Duration of a Trial of Therapy

Published literature indicates that an adequate trial with a standard neuroleptic is a minimum of six weeks. Considering its significance, the shortage of data on this issue is remarkable. Clozapine appears exceptional in this context, in that there is compelling data suggesting that improvement continues to occur throughout a six-month trial period (Meltzer et al 1989). A recent study observed maximum responses to clozapine at 10 months, suggesting that a trial of 9 to 12 months should be conducted before concluding that there is no response to the drug (Jalenques, Albuisson and Tauveron 1996). In a disease where relapse rates may be as high as 50% in two years (Crow et al 1986), several studies involving long-term follow-up with clozapine have demonstrated continuing benefit in terms of sustained initial improvement and prevention of relapse (Lindstrom 1988; Leppig et al 1989; Kuha and Miettinen 1986).

Newer Agents

Clinical evidence suggests that *sulpiride*, an antipsychotic agent with affinity for dopamine D2, D3 and D4 receptors, has similar efficacy to conventional antipsychotics in the treatment of acute schizophrenia (Caley and Weber 1995). There are no data supporting effectiveness in the long-term treatment of schizophrenia or in the treatment of negative symptoms of schizophrenia. While major responses are evident by 6–8 weeks, one extended duration trial of sulpiride continued to show improvement up to 12 weeks (Gerlach et al 1985).

Risperidone is a well-tolerated antipsychotic agent combining potent serotonin (5HT2)and dopamine D2 receptor antagonism. Although trials have not been published specifically addressing the efficacy of risperidone in treatment-resistant schizophrenia, it is possible that the drug may be effective in cases where conventional neuroleptics have failed. Evidence from non-comparative and comparative studies in schizophrenia indicate that risperidone achieves maximal responses at 4–8 weeks, and that these responses may be maintained for up to 12 months (Grant and Fitton 1994). There is, however, no suggestion of a continued increase in efficacy beyond 8 weeks, nor is there data regarding longer term clinical outcomes.

Two other new agents, *sertindole* and *ziprasidone*, are similar to risperidone in that their main antagonism is against dopamine (D2), serotonin and noradrenaline. Sertindole is now available clinically, while ziprasidone is still undergoing trial work. Sertindole has an especially low propensity for extrapyramidal side-effects (EPSE), which have been reported at placebo levels in clinical trials, but there is so far no evidence for superior antipsychotic efficacy. Ziprasidone may cause less EPSE than conventional treatments, but similarly appears equivalent to conventional treatments as an antipsychotic.

Other new agents which resemble clozapine in that they bind to multiple receptors (Gerlach and Peacock 1995) include *olanzapine*, *quetiapine* and *zotepine*. *Olanzapine* has just been granted marketing authorisation, while seroquel and zotepine are still under trial.

Olanzapine's receptor binding profile is similar to that of clozapine and, like sertindole, it is reported to induce EPSE at placebo rates. It was found to be superior to haloperidol for negative symptoms in one very large trial with 2000 patients, although it was not found to be superior in positive symptoms (Tollefson et al 1996). The largest study of nearly 600 patients (Hirsch 1994) reported no difference in EPSE between the seroquel, chlorpromazine and placebo groups. The antipsychotic efficacy of seroquel was equivalent to chlorpromazine. *Quetiapine* is primarily a noradrenaline antagonist. *Zotepine* has high affinity for multiple dopamine and serotonin receptors as well as noradrenaline, and one report of 126 patients (Raniwalla et al 1996) found a better effect on negative symptoms than haloperidol, coupled with significantly less EPSE.

The wider choice of new atypical antipsychotics should be useful in the management of treatment-resistant and treatment-intolerant patients. However, none of the new agents has been shown to be clinically equivalent to clozapine in antipsychotic effect. In addition, none has been shown to take longer to achieve full potential efficacy than conventional neuroleptics, unlike clozapine in which full efficacy may develop over several months. It would seem unreasonable to try the full range of six atypical antipsychotics in every patient who did not respond to conventional treatments. A case could be made for giving either risperidone, sertindole or ziprasidone for 6–8 weeks, followed if there is no response by a further 6–8 weeks of either olanzapine, quetiapine or zotepine before trying clozapine. Until more clinical study results are available it is difficult to make a strong case for interposing further lengthy stages in the management of treatment-resistant illness because of the possible deleterious consequences of withholding what may well be the only effective treatment.

Depot Neuroleptic

What constitutes an adequate trial of a depot neuroleptic is unclear. In general, patients would be stabilised on an oral antipsychotic before commencing depot medication. Transfer to depot medication may be difficult because duration of action is poorly understood, several months may be required to reach steady state serum concentrations, and the formulas for converting oral to parenteral doses are variable and often arbitrary. Although trials of efficacy of various depot antipsychotics have ranged in duration from three weeks (Chouinard and Annable 1976) to five years (Youssef 1989), it has been stated that there is no inherent difference in clinical efficacy, when compliance is assured, between depot and oral medications (Davis et al 1994).

Adjunctive Treatments

There is a great volume of literature addressing adjunctive therapies in treatment-resistant schizophrenia, with evidence of efficacy most strongly documented for the benzodiazepines (Wolkowitz and Pickar 1991; Wolkowitz et al 1992; Christison Kirch and Wyatt 1991), lithium (Christison, Kirch and Wyatt 1991; Atre-Vaidya and Taylor 1989) and carbamazepine (Christison, Kirch and Wyatt 1991; Simhandl and Meszaros 1992). Reported response rates of patients with schizophrenia to benzodiazepines have been 30–50%, although the magnitude of the response is typically modest (Wolkowitz and Pickar 1991). Lithium appears to be beneficial in reducing affective symptomatology in people with schizophrenia and may be useful as an adjunct to neuroleptics in selected treatment-resistant patients (Christison, Kirch and Wyatt 1991). Modest benefit in such patients is also possible with the anticonvulsant carbamazepine (Simhandl and Meszaros 1992); however, trials with sodium valproate have been less encouraging (McElroy et al 1989). Finally, electroconvulsive therapy is effective in acute schizophrenia (Varghese and Singh 1985; Martin 1986) but is neither a first choice nor of any proven benefit in chronic illness (Christison, Kirch and Wyatt 1991).

A recent review of adjunctive therapies in schizophrenia finds it difficult to draw conclusions or develop treatment guidelines from the existing literature (Johns and Thompson 1995). Concerns regarding sample sizes and inconsistent study design have made efficacy data difficult to interpret, and it is impossible to make any firm statement regarding the duration of such adjunctive treatments. It seems unlikely that benefit would be gained by continued treatment if no response was observed after 4–6 weeks.

OUTCOMES

Even with early intervention in schizophrenia there may be adverse consequences in biological, psychological and social terms, but delay in treatment is clearly detrimental (Birchwood, McGorry and Jackson 1997). Efforts to enhance the education of health care professionals, particularly with a shift of resources towards primary care, is important. Education for families, de-stigmatising illness, perhaps facilitated by enhanced care outside of hospital settings, may allow for engagement with patients and promote a willingness to accept treatment and advice. On average, the time from first onset of psychotic symptoms to presentation and treatment is one year. Those taking more than one year to access and exit services had a three-fold increase in the relapse rate over the next two years in the Northwick Park study of first episode schizophrenia (Johnstone et al 1986).

The early outcome of schizophrenia in the first two years is a strong predictor of progress over the next decade. In a prospective study of the outcome of patients with first episode schizophrenia in Nottingham over 13 years, 52% were without psychotic symptoms in the last two years of follow-up, 55% were described as having a good to fair level of social function, though only 17% were alive without symptoms or disability and receiving no treatment (Mason 1995). Patients may be refractory to medication with target symptoms not responding to treatment. Patients may be non-compliant with medication or co-morbid conditions such as depression, anxiety, obsessive-compulsive disorder or personality disorder may interfere with the response. Coincidental substance misuse is prevalent in schizophrenic patients, with a 56% rate of substance misuse reported in one study (Shaner et al 1997).

The International Pilot Study of Schizophrenia of the World Health Organisation demonstrated cultural differences with the Aarhus patients showing a 60% prevalence of active psychotic symptoms at five years compared to 34% of patients in Ibadan and Aggra (Leff et al 1992).

CONCLUSION

It is appropriate to take a rigorous approach when defining what constitutes adequate doses and duration of conventional neuroleptics in the severely ill and difficult-to-treat patient. A reasonable consensus statement would suggest that the patient be considered resistant to treatment if substantial improvement was not observed after trials of six weeks or greater duration, of at least two conventional neuroleptics of different classes, at doses up to the equivalent of 40 mg per day of haloperidol or 600-1000 mg per day of chlorpromazine. However, in the absence of any evidence suggesting that one conventional antipsychotic is more effective than any other, use of the second drug where no initial response has been seen is questionable. Many consider that more would be achieved by trying one of the newer neuroleptics, or adding adjunctive treatments, than by prolonging the use of conventional drugs. Whichever approach is used, there is a need for rapid recognition of treatment resistance and the early institution of effective measures.

REFERENCES

Andreasen NC, Arndt S, Alliger R, Miller D & Flaum M (1995) Symptoms of schizophrenia: methods meanings and mechanisms *Arch Gen Psychiat* **52**: 341–51

Atre-Vaidya N & Taylor MA (1989) Effectiveness of lithium in schizophrenia: Do we really have an answer? *J Clin Psychiat* **50**: 170–2

Birchwood M, McGorry P & Jackson H (1997) Early intervention in schizophrenia *Br J Psychiat* **170**: 2–5

Brenner HD & Merlo MCG (1995) Definition of therapy-resistant schizophrenia and its assessment *Eur Psychiat* **10** (supp 1): 11–17

Caley CF & Weber SS (1995). Sulpiride: an antipsychotic with selective dopaminergic antagonist properties. *Ann Pharmacother* **29**: 152–60

Chouinard G & Annable L (1976) Penfluridol in the treatment of newly admitted schizophrenic patients in a brief therapy unit *Am J Psychiat* **133**: 7

Christison GW, Kirch DG & Wyatt RJ (1991) When symptoms persist: choosing among alternative somatic treatments for schizophrenia *Schizophrenia Bull* **17**(2): 217–45

Crow TJ, MacMillan JF, Johnson A & Johnston E (1986) The Northwick Park study of first episodes of schizophrenia 2 *Br J Psychiat* **148**: 120–7

Davis JM (1980) Important issues in the drug treatment of schizophrenia *Schizophrenia Bull* **6**: 70–87

Davis JM, Metalon L, Watanabe MD & Blake L (1994) Depot antipsychotic drugs: place in therapy *Drugs* **47**(5): 741–73

Gerlach J, Behnke K, Hetberg J, Munk-Andersen C & Neilsen H (1985) Sulpiride and haloperidol in schizophrenia: a double-blind cross-over study of therapeutic effect, side effects and plasma concentrations *Br J Psychiat* **147**: 283–8

Gerlach J & Peacock L (1995) New antipsychotics: the present status *Internat Clin Psychopharmacol* **10** (supp 3): 39–48

Grant S & Fitton A (1994) Risperidone: a review of its pharmacology and therapeutic potential in the treatment of schizophrenia *Drugs* **48**(2): 253–73

Healy D (1991) D1 and D2 and D3 *Br J Psychiat* **159**: 319–24

Hollister LE, Overall JE, Imbell I & Pokorny A (1974) Specific indications for different classes of phenothiazines *Arch Gen Psychiat* **30**: 94–9

Hirsch SR (1986) Clinical treatment of schizophrenia. In PB Bradley & ST Hirsch (eds) *The Psychopharmacology and Treatment of Schizophrenia* Oxford University Press: Oxford

Hirsch SR (1994) Seroquel: an example of an atypical antipsychotic drug *Neuropsychopharmacology* **10** (supp 3): 371S

Huckle PL & Palia SS (1993) Managing resistant schizophrenia *Br J Hosp Med* **50**: 467–71

Jalenques I, Albuisson E & Tauveron I (1996) Clozapine in treatment-resistant schizophrenic patients; preliminary results from an open prospective study *Irish J Psychol Med* **13**(1): 13–18

Jeste DV, Caliguiri MP, Paulsen JS, Heaton RK, Lacro JP, Harris MJ, Bailey A & Fell RL (1995) Risks of tardive dyskinesia in older patients: a prospective longitudinal study of 266 outpatients *Arch Gen Psychiat* 756–65

Johns CA & Thompson JW (1995) Adjunctive treatments in schizophrenia: pharmacotherapies and electroconvulsive therapy *Schizophrenia Bull* **21**(4): 607–19

Johnson DAW (1988) Drug treatment of schizophrenia. In Bebbington & McGuffin (eds) *Schizophrenia the Major Issues* Heineman Professional Publishing: Oxford

Johnstone EC, Crow TJ, Johnson AL et al (1986) The Northwick Park study of first episode, schizophrenia 1 *Br J Psychiat* **148**: 115–20

Kane J, Honigfeld G, Singer J & Meltzer H (1988) Clozapine for the treatment-resistant schizophrenic; a double blind comparison with chlorpromazine *Arch Gen Psychiat* **45**: 789–96

Keefe RS, Lobel DS, Mohs RC, Silverman JM, Harvey PD, Davidson M, Losonczy MF & Davis KL (1991) Diagnostic issues in chronic schizophrenia: Kraepelinian schizophrenia, undifferentiated schizophrenia, and state-independent negative symptoms *Schizophrenia Res* **4**(2): 71–9

King DJ (1990) The effects of neuroleptics on cognitive and psychomotor functioning *Br J Psychiat* **157**: 799–811

Kohen D & Bristow M (1996) Neuroleptic malignant syndrome *Adv Psychiat Treat* **2**: 151–7

Kuha S & Miettinen E (1986) Long term effect of clozapine in schizophrenia: a retrospective study of 108 chronic schizophrenics treated with clozapine for up to 7 years *Nord Psykiatr Tidssk* **40**: 225–30

Leff J, Sartorius N, Jableusky A, Korten A & Ernberg G (1992) The international pilot study of schizophrenia: five year follow-up of findings *Psychol Med* **22**: 131–45

Leppig M, Bosch B, Naber D & Hippius H (1989) Clozapine in the treatment of 121 outpatients *Psychopharmacol* **9** (supp): 77–9

Lewander T (1992) Differential development of therapeutic drugs for psychosis. *Clin Neuropharmacol* **15** (supp 1): 654–5

Lieberman JA, Mayerhoff D, Loebel A, Degreef C, Levy D & Alvir J (1991) Biologic indices of heterogeneity in schizophrenia: relationship to psychopathology and treatment outcome *Schizophrenia Res* **4**: 289–90

Lindstrom LH (1988) The effect of long term treatment of clozapine in schizophrenia: a retrospective study of 96 patients treated with clozapine for up to 13 years *Acta Psychiatrica* **77**: 524–9

Livingston MG (1994) Risperidone *Lancet* **343**: 457–60

Martin BA (1986) Electroconvulsive therapy: contemporary standards of practice *Can J Psychiatry* **31**: 759–71

Mason P (1995) Characteristic of outcome in schizophrenia at 13 years *Br J Psychiat* 596–603

McElroy SL, Keck PE, Pope HC Jr & Hudson JI (1989) Valproate in psychiatric disorders: literature review and clinical guidelines *J Clin Psychiat* **50** (supp 3): 23–9

Meltzer HY, Bastani B, Kwon KY, Ramirex LF, Burnett S & Sharpe J (1989) A prospective study of clozapine in treatment-resistant schizophrenic patients, I: preliminary report *Psychopharmacol* **9** (supp): 68–72

Meltzer HY (1992) Treatment of the neuroleptic-non-responsive schizophrenic patient *Schizophrenia Bull* **18**(3): 515–42

Raniwalla J, Tweed JA, Dollfus S & Petit M (1996) A comparison of an atypical (zotepine) and classical (haloperidol) antipsychotic in patients with acute exacerbation of schizophrenia. *Schizophrenia Res* **2**(3): 133

Rifkin A, Doddi S, Karajgi B, Burenstein M & Wachspress M (1991) Dosage of haloperidol for schizophrenia *Arch Gen Psychiat* **48**: 166–70

Seeman P (1992) Dopamine receptor sequences. Therapeutic levels of neuroleptics occupy D2 receptors, clozapine occupies D4 *Neuropsychopharmacol* **7**: 261–84

Simhandl C & Meszaros K (1992) The use of carbamazepine in the treatment of schizophrenic and schizoaffective psychoses: a review *J Psychiat Neurosci* **17**: 1–14

Shaner A, Khalsa MF, Roberts JL, Wilkins J, Anglin D & Hsieh SC (1997) Unrecognised cocaine abuse among schizophrenic patients *AM J Psychiat* **150**: 758–62

Stahl SM & Wets KM (1988) Recent advances in drug delivery technology for neurology *Clin Neuropharmacol* **11**: 1–17

Tollefson GD, Beasley CM, Tran PV, Tamura RN, Sanger T, Wood A & Beuzen JN (1996) Olanzapine versus haloperidol: results of the multicentre international trial *Schizophrenia Res* **2**(3): 131

Varghese FTN & Singh BS (1985) Electroconvulsive therapy in 1985 – a review *Med J Austral* **143**: 192–6

Wolkowitz OM & Pickar D (1991) Benzodiazepines in the treatment of schizophrenia: a review and reappraisal *Am J Psychiat* **148**: 714–26

Wolkowitz OM, Turetsky MA, Reus VI & Hargreaves WA (1992) Benzodiazepine augmentation of neuroleptics in treatment-resistant schizophrenia *Psychopharmacol Bull* **28**(3): 291–5

Youssef HA (1989) A five year follow-up study of chronic schizophrenics and other psychotics treated in the community: depot haloperidol decanoate versus other neuroleptics *Adv Therapeut* **64**: 186–95

Index